OVERCOMING
PAIN

OVERCOMING PAIN

ALLAN PLATT, PA-C
SUSAN PLATT, M.D.
CATHY HEDRICH, RPT

Hilton Publishing Company • CHICAGO, ILLINOIS

Hilton Publishing Company, Inc.
Chicago, Illinois

Direct all correspondence to:
Hilton Publishing Company
110 Ridge Road
Munster, IN 46321
815–885–1070
www.hiltonpub.com

Library of Congress Cataloging-in-Publication Data

Platt, Allan F.
    Overcoming Pain / Allan Platt, Susan Platt, Cathy Hedrich.
        p. cm.
    ISBN 0–9743144-2–0 (pbk. : alk. paper)
    1. Pain—Popular works. I. Platt, Susan, 1956– II. Hedrich, Cathy, 1960–
III. Title.
    RB127.P56 2004
    616'.0472—dc22   2005000766

Printed and bound in the United States of America

CONTENTS

Part Three
THE FUTURE OF PAIN TREATMENT

Part Four
FURTHER RESOURCES

Disclaimer

This book is intended to help patients and their loved ones learn the ABCs of overcoming pain. It is not a substitute for good medical care by a physician. Only your medical care provider can determine if the pain is a warning sign of a serious medical condition.

Dosages and specific medications are only suggestions. The information is not exhaustive and does not cover all ailments, physical conditions, or all their treatments. Only your healthcare provider can know your particular case and design the treatment plan best for you.

FOREWORD

To be human is to know what it is like to have pain. Most of us are fortunate to have the kind of pain that goes away with time and proper treatment. But even our short experiences with pain are enough to convince us that being in pain is, experientially, one of the worst states of being. Now imagine if you had pain everyday, and that your efforts to get help seemed endless—one doctor and treatment after another—and resulted in little relief. That, unfortunately, is the experience of millions of Americans.

There are over 50 million people in the United States living with various kinds of pain. Despite their best efforts, many of these people have not found adequate help for their pain. Part of the explanation for this is that people do not have the information that they need in order to get the best results from the medical care system. In accessing medical help, knowledge is power. In getting help for relieving pain, particularly chronic pain, this is even more true.

Advances in understanding pain have made one thing clear—pain is complex. There are different causes, different mechanisms, different ways in which people respond to similar treatments, different combinations of treatments, different attitudes of patients and providers, and different contexts in which treatment is provided. The complexity begs for clarification and explanation.

Enter *Overcoming Pain*. The authors, Allan Platt, Susan Platt, and Cathy Hedrich, have succeeded in providing a resource that is both comprehensive and simple. It takes the reader through the ABC's of pain, including the basic science of pain, information about the assessing pain, and the ins and outs of the medical system.

The main part of the text discusses the array of treatment options. *Overcoming Pain* displays its virtuosity by its coverage of pain relief "tools," such as meditation, prayer, therapeutic exercise, distraction techniques, yoga, and relaxation therapy. In fact, the book makes clear that just as pain is usually not a simple phenomenon, the best treatment approach is as complex as that pain, involving many approaches—medicine, non-medicines, and attention to cultural, social, emotional, and spiritual aspects of pain. *Overcoming Pain* is also solid in its accounting of the traditional medical tools—medicines, interventions, and devices.

The last section of the book talks about the future of pain treatment. It covers very practical information about living with pain and facing the future. It covers emotional health, understanding race and pain, the nature of clinical trials and how to participate in them, and the importance of pain advocacy.

From the perspective of the person affected by pain, this book will not only be an important read, but an important reference resource. As people search for the combination of elements for their pain management plan, this book can be a guide each time there is a question about which way to turn. A thank you to the authors for providing such an easy-to-read and comprehensive map.

William Rowe,
Executive Director
American Pain Foundation

Part One

THE ABCS OF PAIN

CHAPTER 1

What Pain Is and How It's Best Treated

WHY WE HAVE PAIN

If you are reading this book because you are experiencing pain, it may be hard for us to convince you that pain has its uses. In fact, it has several. Pain is a kind of alarm system that warns you of a danger to your body or to your health.

For example, when you touch a hot stove, you feel a sharp pain, and your body reacts by withdrawing quickly from the stove to prevent further damage.

When you have a headache because you feel overstressed, pain is warning you to calm down. It can also tell you that you have sprained your ankle or stepped on a nail, or, by way of chest pains called angina, tell you that your heart is starved for blood. Such pain, in brief, can be an urgent reason to see your doctor.

> *Pain is a kind of alarm system that warns you of a danger to your body or to your health.*

Only the person experiencing a pain can know how it feels and how often it comes back. By describing these as exactly as you can, you help your physician to diagnose problems. In some cases, continuing high intensity of pain may be a lifesaving alarm signaling that you need an operation.

Pain is so important to us that people with diabetes, who don't feel pain because of nerve damage, can injure themselves—say, by stepping on a sharp object and not feeling a thing. Such numbness to pain can lead to serious infection and body damage.

But while pain is a good warning system, it's not perfect. Sometimes the system's wires get crossed, and they signal pain when there is no reason to. Such pain can last for days, months, and years. Chronic pain can take away your ability to relax, work, enjoy, or function. But there *is* good news. While your doctor may not be able to completely ease your pain, he or she, with the help of a good health team, can teach you to manage pain so that you suffer less.

But there is good news. While your doctor may not always be able to cure your pain, he or she, with the help of a good health team, can teach you to manage pain so that you suffer less.

There is also a lot you can do for yourself. This book is meant to be a toolbox for your use. People who understand pain are most likely to get good treatment and support. That's why you must be an educated consumer, and the aim of *Overcoming Pain* is to make you one. No one should be overcome by pain.

WHY PAIN MATTERS

Statistically, we know the following:

- Pain is the most common reason for medical appointments in the United States (140 million visits a year).

- $100 billion each year goes to health costs and lost work time (50 million lost workdays each year).
- 48 million Americans experience chronic pain.
- 21.6 million are on routine pain medications.

But statistics can only show so much. The most important fact is that chronic pain has a great impact on the lives of people who have to cope with it.

Some of the ways pain can affect you:

- It can interfere with your sleep.
- It can cut down your appetite.
- It can lessen your activity.
- It can keep you from work.
- It can force you to drop hobbies and recreation.
- It can weaken your immune system's ability to fight infections.
- It can mean spending days in a hospital bed.

One important problem we address in this book is that, in far too many cases, the medical establishment under treats pain. An American Pain Society study found that four out of ten people who have chronic pain not related to cancer don't get relief below 5 on a 0 to 10 pain scale. That means a lot of people are walking around with a lot of pain.

A key reason why 47 percent of people with pain have changed doctors at least once and 22 percent have switched three or more times is because many people don't get adequate relief. When they were asked for reasons why they changed doctors, 37 percent said that their doctors didn't know enough about pain, 29 percent said their doctors didn't take their pain seriously enough, and 27 percent found their doctors unwilling to treat it aggressively.

"This is a great country to be sick in, but not a great country to have pain in. We have excellent high-tech medicine,
and if you want to be cured, this is where you want to be.
But if you are in a lot of pain that's never going to go away,
it would be better to be in England, Germany, Japan, or
any of the Scandinavian countries."

—Bill Moyers, *On Our Own Terms: Moyers on Dying*
PBS, September, 2000

WHY PAIN IS UNDER TREATED

Pain is not treated very effectively because:

- It is hard to measure.
- Doctors get little training about pain in medical school.
- There are few centers for treating pain.

Because pain *is* hard to measure, pain is what you say it is.
Everyone experiences pain a little differently. In our age of MRI
scans and blood tests, the fact that
they have no tests to measure pain
but must rely on your word makes
many doctors nervous, and therefore
more ready to discount or downgrade
your own estimation of the pain.

> *Because pain is
> hard to measure,
> pain is what you
> say it is.*

Another reason why pain is under
treated is that it is underreported by
patients. Many people fear they will be seen as complainers if they
ask for pain medication. In fact, some cultures encourage this atti-
tude, and *do* see it as a sign of weakness to talk about pain.

PAIN AND MINORITIES

If you are in a minority ethnic group, you are more likely to be under treated for pain, even if you come into the emergency room with, say, a fracture. Pharmacies in minority neighborhoods aren't always very helpful, either. They may not even stock certain pain medications because of fear of robbery. Further, we are sad to say, minority patients under use hospice services that could help relieve pain at the end of life.

Ensuring that minority patients get the best possible treatment is no easy task, given the complexity of the issues. Racism also comes to bear, so there are doctors who adequately treat White patients but under treat Blacks or Latinos.

The fact is, doctors aren't comfortable talking with patients, Black or White, about pain, and, even after the pain has been diagnosed, they're uncomfortable talking about treatment options. Nurses, too, sometimes add to the problem by under medicating a patient, even though they've received a prescription for higher doses. The upshot is that many people are under treated and must live with their pain every day.

A special aspect of the issue is that the medical establishment is especially fearful about using opiate medications, our most potent weapon against pain. They worry about drug addiction, and they also worry about a government agency investigating whether they're prescribing what the agency considers too many opiates.

You can see that a great deal of fear and misunderstanding surrounds the problem of pain.

WHAT IS BEING DONE?

You've heard the bad news. But there is also good news for people who suffer with pain. The medical system is starting to take pain more seriously, and studies are going on to find ways to measure and treat pain more accurately and effectively. Finally, the Joint Commission on the Accreditation of Healthcare Organizations (JCAHO) has published new pain standards to be complied with by the entire medical establishment, including nursing homes.

The JCAHO pain standards require healthcare facilities to do the following:

- Recognize the right of patients to receive assessment and treatment of pain.
- Inform patients about pain and pain relief options.
- Believe and respond quickly to patients' reports of pain.
- Ensure that patients have access to state-of-the-art pain management and pain relief specialists.
- Assess the intensity of pain—the assessment to include:
  - Locating the pain.
  - Determining associated symptoms, environment, onset, duration, timing, and conditions and medications that make pain better or worse.
  - Determining how well the patient functions, past history, physical examination, and severity of the pain as measured by a valid scale.
  - Recording the pain assessment in a way that lays the groundwork for regular reassessment and follow-up.

All of the above procedures must be documented and tracked over time. If there is more than one site of pain, each site needs this documentation.

The recommendations go still further. Medical institutions are asked to educate and test medical staff about pain assessment and pain management. This education is to include:

- What causes pain.
- Pain assessment methods.

- Medications to treat pain.
- Non-medication treatments.

The recommendations also ask that medical institutions establish policies and procedures that support good pain treatment, educate patients and their families about good pain treatment, and provide good pain treatment at home after the patient leaves the hospital.

These standards are endorsed by the American Pain Society (*www.ampainsoc.org*) which recommends that pain be included as the fifth vital sign examining doctors should look for in assessing the health of your body (the other vital signs are body temperature, pulse, respiration rate, and blood pressure).

PAIN MEDICINE—A NEW SPECIALTY

There is a growing new specialty in medicine under the leadership of physicians with special training in pain management. There are now pain clinics with medical staff dedicated to the many needs of people with everyday pain. It is now understood that pain can be attacked from many levels—with medications, blocks, surgery, special pumps, nerve stimulation, behavior changes, special diets, relaxation, physical therapy, job rehabilitation, education, and distraction. New research is opening new treatment avenues and also helping us better understand the causes and the prevention of chronic pain.

HELPING YOURSELF

Pain treatment education is now entering the medical and nursing schools, so we will have a better-equipped medical system. But there are also things you must do on your own behalf. People who suffer from chronic pain need to become educated consumers who know their rights as patients, and who understand what treatments are available to them.

In *Overcoming Pain,* we aim to take away the mystery that still surrounds pain, and to inspire hope to replace fear. As you read, you will learn:

- The causes of pain.
- The types of pain.
- How to measure pain.
- Your treatment options.
- How to cope with special challenges associated with pain.
- How to make informed decisions about treatment options.
- How to deal with the medical world.

In addition, *Overcoming Pain* gives you a list of resources that can provide you with both information and support.

Pain Matters

Overcoming Pain is meant to be a working toolbox to help you win the struggle against pain rather than being overwhelmed by it.

CHAPTER 2

How Pain Works
in the Body

In this chapter, we'll tell you about how pain works in the body and how you can make it less intense (or even go away) and easier to cope with. Acting on this knowledge, you can face your ordinary, daily life with new strength and confidence.

AT THE TISSUE LEVEL

Your finger slips across the sharp edge of a knife while you are cutting up an apple. The knife not only slices through your skin, but it has also cut several nerve endings and small blood vessels. At the site of the wound, cells break apart, releasing chemicals that activate the nerve to send a message that damage has occurred.

THE WIRING SYSTEM

The pain message races through the network of nerves to the main trunk of all the body's wiring, the spinal cord, before the first drop of blood oozes from the cut. The spinal cord acts as a switch box and relay station to send the message upward to the brain on a fast track.

Any damage to the spinal cord can cause lack of feeling below the injured area. If you have had the kind of fall that causes the discs that pad the backbone to push on the nerves entering the spinal cord, you may experience numbness in the area supplied by that nerve, or shooting pains down the arms or legs.

THE BRAIN AS CONTROL BOX

The pain message from the finger also races up the spinal cord and enters the Grand Central Station of all the nerve endings, the brain. In the case of the knife cut, the pain message is now directed to the area of the brain that receives messages from the hands and fingers. Because this knife cut sliced more nerves than, say, a pinprick would, the message is more intense.

The brain mobilizes its defenses quickly, within a second of the slice, and a complex message, which instantly becomes action, goes to many parts of your body. Messages go out to the arm, hand, and finger muscles to withdraw from the knife to prevent further injury. Other messages, to the nerves that control the muscles of the cut finger, cause them to contract. Even your mouth and vocal chords are part of this alarm system. Messages from them make you shout "Ouch!" Other messages help block the pain messages coming up from the wounded finger.

While this is going on, your eyes focus on the cut, where a drop of blood is forming, and your finger pulls away from the knife. Your right hand now grabs the injured finger to put pressure on the cut. Your pain is decreased by the sensation of fingers squeezing the wounded site. Your mind is distracted as you look for a bandage to cover the wound. This decreases the sharp pain even more.

A few minutes later, with the bandage in place, the finger wound begins to throb as damaged cells release chemicals and the damaged blood vessels leak fluid into the surrounding area. Repair work begins to close the sliced skin and remove the damaged cells. All this happens in an instant, most of it invisible to you except in the results.

OUR RESPONSES TO PAIN

Each of us responds in a different way to the pain of a sliced finger. Some will scream, others faint, curse, jump up and down, or simply cover the cut without fuss. All sorts of things bear on the way you respond to pain, such as:

- Age.
- Cultural background.
- How you were taught as a child to deal with pain.
- Your ability to endure pain.
- Your knowledge about pain and its causes.
- Your mood at the time (depression or fear makes pain worse).

Distracting your brain from the pain is an important part of your toolbox. Different people will find different ways to do this. Common distractions are:

- Music.
- Relaxation.
- Physical activity.
- Reading.
- Video games.
- Hobbies.

To understand the importance of distraction, consider how an athlete injured in sports games may continue playing with minimal pain because his or her mind is focused on playing the game. The pain will become intense only later, when the mind is not focused on other things. Thinking about pain increases it, just as the volume control on the radio makes it louder.

PAIN IS WHAT YOU SAY IT IS

We experience pain in the hidden parts of the brain and nervous system that medical devices can't scan. That's why pain is what you say it is. What's a mild pain for you may feel like extreme pain to another person with the same injury.

That means that your doctor must hear you describe the pain to get clues about how to treat it. Communication between you and your doctor is most important. This means that your doctor must know how to listen, but it also means that you must know how to describe the pain exactly, in a way your doctor can understand.

Pain Matters

Pain is what you say it is. You can help yourself by understanding how pain serves as a red light warning system of injury or disease. In some cases, pain that begins for a specific cause continues even when the healing process is successful. Knowing the cause of your pain is an important part of your getting the most effective treatment.

CHAPTER 3

Types of Pain

Devarius was driving home from work when another car ran a red light and broadsided his car. His air bag and seat belt kept him from serious injury, but he had a wide collection of bumps, bruises, and aches across his body. Even now, four months later, Devarius still wakes up stiff and sore, and has times when he cannot turn his head without pain.

Shawna cannot remember the exact day she started having what she calls "body aches," but she thinks it may have started with a bad case of the flu. Some days she only has muscle soreness in her legs; on other days she is in such pain she cannot get out of bed. Cold weather and stress make her pain worse, and nothing she has tried permanently stops the pain.

Mario was playing a pick-up game of basketball at the gym. Going up for a rebound, he was knocked off balance and landed awkwardly on his ankle. The game was tied, and he kept playing despite the pain. Now his ankle is so swollen he can't get his shoe on. It hurts Mario to walk, and he has developed a limp.

For the treatment of pain, as for pain itself, there is no "one size that fits all." Because pain can have so many different causes (accident, injury, surgery or disease), people perceive and respond to pain in different ways. A nagging headache to one person may be an awful migraine to another. Even finding effective treatment that relieves pain differs from patient to patient. A particular treatment that relieves pain for one person may actually increase pain in another.

And if those different possible types and treatments of pain aren't enough, weather, activity, stress, and fatigue can cause a person to feel more pain.

But despite all those differences in how people feel pain, there *is* one constant: No one wants to be in pain that goes on and on, through weeks and months and even years.

ACUTE, SUB-ACUTE, AND CHRONIC PAIN

How long a pain has been going on is one of the ways that doctors determine the best treatment for it. Pain can be divided into three levels: acute, sub-acute, and chronic pain. Each level has different characteristics, but what they have in common is that they undermine one's physical, mental, and emotional well-being.

Acute pain: This pain occurs suddenly, often as a result of injury or surgery. Acute pain tends to be continuous. It can range from mild to severe. Bruising, redness, swelling, muscle spasms, and tenderness are often present, and moving usually makes the pain worse. Acute pain can last up to one month and almost always responds well to treatment. As the injured area of the body heals, the pain lessens day by day until it is gone.

Sub-acute pain: This is less severe than acute pain, but it stays around longer and has occasional "spikes" of increased intensity. Activity, stress, and tiredness can make sub-acute pain worse, while movement may decrease it. A person with sub-acute pain may experience muscle spasms, tenderness, and swelling. This type of pain can last for anywhere from two to six months. Sub-acute pain usually responds well to treatment.

Chronic pain: This is a steady pain that lasts longer than six months. In the case of chronic pain, nervous system wiring becomes over sensitive to normal signals and sends them to the brain as pain messages. There may be no signs of body damage that could cause the pain, but the pain is there and it is real. Chronic pain may get better for a while, then worse, in an endless cycle, sometimes limiting a person's activity and ability to function normally. A person with chronic pain may experience muscle spasms, tenderness, and hypersensitivity, individually or together.

Chronic pain is the most challenging to treat, but it can be managed by treating pain early in the acute phase.

Chronic pain can have several repercussions on your health. For one, with the onset of chronic pain, a downward spiral of limited mobility and inability to carry on your normal activities begins. A second repercussion is that pain causes muscle spasms. Finally, pain causes a behavior called "guarding," which means that a patient will avoid using the injured part for fear of added pain. Guarding further limits movement and increases pain.

The upshot of this is an overall loss of strength that can lead to the inability to tolerate *any* activity. What follows is severe confinement to a chair or bed, along with more and more pain.

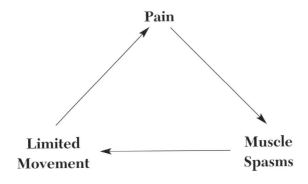

To break this cycle, the first job is to reduce the level of pain. Once pain is under control, a patient can regain movement and slowly build strength. Step by step, the patient will begin to be able to get back to the regular activities that severe pain has made impossible. But this can't happen if pain is allowed to continue untreated.

CAUSES OF PAIN

Injury

Pain from an injury usually has an obvious cause—a cut, scrape, broken bone, or burn. Pain caused by an injury is usually felt immediately, but there is also a secondary pain in the injured area as it repairs. "Healing pain" can be severe, depending on the size of the injury and the number of nerves reporting pain to the brain. Individual nerves can be injured or damaged cells release chemicals that cause the nerves to send the pain message to the brain. Pain caused by an injury is usually described as sharp and intense.

Common types of injury pain include:

- Low back strain.
- Sprained ankles.
- Tennis elbow.
- Any muscle strain from misuse or overuse.

Surgery is a planned body injury, or cut, to repair or remove something. Doctors use medicine to make you numb or sleep so deeply that you do not feel pain. After the surgery, when the medicine wears off, you may need pain medication to help you heal.

Inflammation

After an injury has occurred, inflammation takes over, as the body starts the repair process. The blood vessels leak fluid into the injured area, and white blood cells invade to clean up germs and dead cells. When cells break apart, they release chemicals that cause the blood flow to increase and the blood vessels to leak. More white blood cells are called to come to the area. That whole process is behind what we call "inflammation."

The inflamed area will be swollen, warmer, and redder than the surrounding area. Nerves in the inflamed area send pain signals back to the brain. This kind of pain is usually described as "throbbing."

Anti-inflammatory medicines, which help block inflammation, are usually part of pain treatment.

No Flow, No Go

When blood flow is blocked for any reason, such as a blood clot or sickled red cells, the cells downstream from the blockage starve from a lack of oxygen and begin to die, releasing chemicals that cause both inflammation and injury pain. This pain can be mild at first, but as more cells die from lack of oxygen, the pain grows in intensity. The outside skin of an area with blocked blood flow may first look pale and then inflamed, as cells die and the repair process begins.

Pain caused by blockage of the blood vessels can also be the deep, squeezing, and chest tightness of angina, which is caused by decreased blood flow to the heart muscle. Or it can be the sharp pain in the legs called "claudication," which happens when a person with a blockage exercises his or her legs.

If a person is confined to bed for a long time, a blood clot can form in the calf or thigh, and then break off and float to the lungs, where it blocks blood flow to an area. The result is what doctors call a *pulmonary embolus* or PE. PE causes sharp chest pain with each breath. Should you experience such a pain call your doctor or 911 emergency services at once. The key to treating PE is to get the blood flowing again.

Nerves Gone Wild

Some diseases, like diabetes, damage the nerves so that they carry the wrong message. The nerves transmit a burning sensation where there is no skin damage. This is called "neuropathic pain." The nerve damage may eventually block all feeling in the area supplied by the nerve, so that the patient will no longer experience the "good pain" that normally alerts us to cuts, bites, burns, and punctures.

In the beginning stages of this nerve damage, patients experience a shooting or burning sensation that can be very annoying. Traditional pain medications may not work against this very bothersome feeling. Patients often find more effective treatment in the antiseizure medicines that help stabilize nerves in the brain, and in certain types of antidepressant medications.

Another common way nerves can be damaged is by pressure from a disc or bone spur that pushes on the nerve. This kind of nerve damage starts when the discs begin to bulge as the result of aging or back injury or when bone spurs develop over time. Such pain is treated with anti-inflammatory medication and, if necessary, by surgery to remove the bone pressure on the nerve.

Stretching

Many organs inside the body, including the liver, intestines, and spleen, have nerves that sense stretching of the organ. When these organs do stretch and grow in size because of disease, there is a feeling of deep interior pain hard to pinpoint or locate. You may have had the sensation from too much gas in your intestines, which caused stomach pain that went away when the gas passed. This is called "visceral pain." Visceral pains that *don't* go away may be the first clue to something going wrong on the inside, and need a doctor's attention.

Invasion

When cancer invades a body part or organ, it can damage normal cells and nerves and irritate stretched nerves. The result can be intense pain in the bones, organs, or nerves. Such pain, called "invasion pain," is a combination of all of the types of pain described above.

Other causes of invasion pain are infections from something as common as a tooth abscess, or a strep throat that causes tonsil swelling and pain. More serious infections like HIV and tuberculosis, or TB, can invade bones and organs, causing deep pain where cells are damaged.

PAIN LONG AFTER THE INSULT

Pain from any of the causes listed above can eventually cause "memory" in the nerve system—that is, the sensation of pain long after the insult, injury, or invasion. Memory happens if the pain is not adequately treated early and the signals keep repeating through the nerve wiring system. This repetition leads to chronic pain—that is, pain that last longer than six months. The result can be severe disability that interferes with normal life. Pain experts and pain clinics may be most helpful in breaking the pain cycle.

Pain Matters

Your doctor, with your help, must know the type of pain you're experiencing in order to find the right treatment. Treatment for chronic pain is different from treatment of the acute pain that results from a fresh injury. The more precisely you can describe the kind of pain you are experiencing, the better your doctor can diagnose and treat it.

CHAPTER 4

The Causes
of Pain

My back is filled with searing pain;
there is no health in my body.

—PSALM 38:7

We've talked about types of pain, and now we turn to their causes. This chapter will give you:

- An overview of the diseases that cause pain.
- An outline of treatments specific to the disease that can reduce pain.
- The information you need in order to find the best type of medical specialist for your particular disease.
- The websites of agencies that can help you find your way out of pain and that point you to further information about your disease.

Remember that the treatment overviews are meant to help you to discuss your condition and treatment with your doctor. They should never substitute for a face-to-face evaluation by your doctor, followed by a discussion between you and your doctor about the best possible treatment options.

INJURIES CAUSED BY ACCIDENT OR BY SURGERY

Injury to the skin, bones, and organs can result from accidents or from surgery. Either way, pain occurs because nerves and cells have been injured and the repair process has begun. Because inflammation is a part of the repair process, this pain will last for several days.

First-level pain treatments and medications will offer relief. These are:

- Cold therapy with ice or cold packs.
- Elevation of the injured area to prevent swelling.
- Use of anti-inflammatory pain medications.

Later, heat therapy will provide pain relief.

JOINT PAIN OR ARTHRITIS

There are two major types of arthritis. The more common is called "osteoarthritis" (*osteo* means "bone"). The less common type is caused by what is called an "autoimmune response"—that is, the body attacks itself, mainly in the joints.

Osteoarthritis results from the everyday wear and tear on the joints as we grow older. It usually affects the fingers, back, neck, knees, and shoulders. The pain ordinarily increases as you use the affected joint.

This type of pain is best treated with first-level pain treatments, then by joint injections that may offer temporary relief, and, eventually, by joint replacement surgery.

Another arthritic joint pain can occur when urate or calcium crystals form in joint fluid to cause a painful arthritis. Usually this happens in the big toe or in the knees. This condition is called *gout* if the crystals are urate, or *pseudogout* if the crystals are calcium. Both respond very well to NSAID (nonsteroidal anti-inflammatory) therapy. Additional treatment, in the form of diet changes or medication, may be needed to prevent further formation of crystals.

Autoimmune type arthritis, caused by the body attacking itself, is made up of many diagnoses, such as:

- Rheumatoid arthritis.
- Psoriatic arthritis.
- Reiter's syndrome.
- Ulcerative bowel disease.
- Systemic Lupus Erythematosis (SLE).

This class of arthritis, when mild, is treated with first-level pain treatments. For second-tier treatment, there are specific medications that may quiet the immune system and prevent it from attacking itself. These medications require careful monitoring and are best prescribed by arthritis experts (Rheumatologists).

For more information, visit the Arthritis Foundation web site at *www.arthritis.org*.

BACK AND NECK PAIN

Back and neck pain can be caused by muscle strain, a slipped disc, arthritis of the bones in the back, or by problems within the body that make the pain travel to the back. The most common cause is muscle strain, which can be treated with first-level pain measures. The internal causes include kidney infections, cancer in the bones, and, rarely, bone infections.

Special exercises for back support and special prevention tricks can help you avoid future back troubles. Work with your primary-care doctor to find out the cause of the problem. Later, if the pain doesn't go away, you may need the services of an orthopedic surgeon, neurosurgeon, chiropractor, or physical therapist.

For more information see: Spine health at *www.spinehealth. com.*

ANGINA—CHEST PAIN

Angina is a feeling of chest heaviness or tightness, or a squeezing pain in the chest, neck, jaw, and left-arm area. Angina often occurs when a person is exercising or exerting themselves, and during periods of stress. It is caused by blocked blood flow to the main blood vessels supplying oxygen to the heart muscle that pumps your blood. Such blockage can result from being overweight, having uncontrolled diabetes, having untreated high blood pressure, or not exercising regularly. Angina is a warning sign that a complete blockage may occur, causing a heart attack. A visit to your primary-care doctor or emergency room is advised immediately.

Treatments includes taking a daily baby aspirin to prevent blood clotting, and nitroglycerine tablets if the chest pain occurs. Nitroglycerine tablets open the blood vessels and increase blood flow to the oxygen-starved muscles. Your doctor also may recommend other prescription medicines.

If you experience angina, your doctor will arrange your visit to the cardiologist (heart specialist) for special tests to see if the blockage can be best managed by medication, by the use of a special catheter and balloon (angioplasty), or by open heart (bypass) surgery.

Other problems that can also cause chest pain include:

- Acid reflux.
- Stomach ulcers.
- Gastritis.
- Gall stones.

- Lung infection or blood clots.
- Irritation (as in shingles).
- Muscle and bone tenderness.

To prevent blood vessel blockage and angina from happening, avoid being overweight, control diabetes, treat high blood pressure, and exercise regularly.

For more information see the American Heart Association at *www.americanheart.org*.

> *To prevent blood vessel blockage and angina from happening, avoid being overweight, control diabetes, treat high blood pressure, and exercise regularly.*

TMJ PAIN—PAIN IN THE JAW

TMJ (temporomandibular joint) pain is an annoying or nagging jaw pain felt in the joint just in front of the ear. This kind of jaw pain can best be evaluated and treated by your dentist or oral surgeon. It is usually caused by grinding your teeth or by jaw misalignment. First-line pain treatment will help relieve the symptoms. (For more on front-line treatment, see Chapter 7.)

For more information see the TMJ Association at *www.tmj.org*.

DIABETES AND NERVE PAIN

Poorly controlled diabetes, over time, can cause nerve damage and pain (neuropathic pain). Typically, this pain is shooting or burning pain. Neuropathic pain can be very annoying, keeping people awake at night, and causing a great deal of discomfort.

There are a number of possible treatments for neuropathic pain, but the best choice varies from person to person. The most commonly effective treatments are anti-seizure (epilepsy) medications, or certain kinds of antidepressants. The doctor who is an expert in diabetes is called an "Endocrinologist," but many primary-care doctors manage this disease well. A consultation with a Neurologist, or nerve expert, may be needed if the pain remains severe.

For more information see the American Diabetes Association at *www.diabetes.org*.

SICKLE CELL DISEASE

Sickle cell disease is in inherited hemoglobin problem that causes red blood cells to become crescent shaped, blocking blood flow in various body parts. Sickle cell is most common in people of African heritage, although it is also found in Greeks, Italians, Saudi Arabians, and people from India, South America, and the Caribbean.

Sickle cell disease can cause intense pain in any part of the body once the sickled red cells start to block blood flow and oxygen. Over time, bone and organ damage can occur, causing daily pain.

Sickle cell disease is best cared for in special clinics with sickle cell experts. Usually the best type of physician is a hematologist with an interest in this disease. A patient can prevent sickle cell pain by drinking plenty of water, keeping well oxygenated, keeping a steady body temperature, and preventing infections. There is also a medication called "hydroxyurea" that actually cuts the number of pain events by half.

For more information see the Sickle Cell Information Center at *www.SCInfo.org*.

HEMOPHILIA

Hemophilia is an inherited condition that only affects males. People with hemophilia lack a factor that helps the blood to clot when you get cut. Hemophilia can cause bleeding into big joints, like the knee, as the result of very minor injuries.

Bleeding in the joints is very painful and requires treatment with a new clotting factor, along with pain treatment. Hematologists or blood specialists are the experts in this disease.

For more information see the National Hemophilia Foundation web site at *www.hemophilia.org*.

HIV

HIV (Human Immunodeficiency Virus) is a viral infection that's carried from person to person by sexual contact, sharing needles, and, rarely, blood transfusion. HIV infection interferes with your body's normal ability to resist infections.

HIV itself does not cause pain, but the infections it brings about, along with the necessary treatments, may cause pain. A brain infection can cause headaches, and infections that appear as rashes can cause skin pain.

Some cancers (for example, Kaposi's sarcoma) and other viral infections (like herpes/shingles) are more common in people with HIV disease.

The medications used to treat the HIV virus can cause nerve damage, leading to the neuropathic pain similar to the pain that affects diabetics.

For more information, see The HIV Insight web site at *www.hivinsite.ucsf.edu*.

HEADACHES

There are many causes of headaches, some of them minor and some life threatening. Causes range from stress and infection, all the way to brain tumors. If you suffer from frequent headaches, see your doctor. If the doctor can't find the cause and your headaches can't be controlled, your doctor may refer you to a Neurologist, or brain expert. The five general categories that cover most, although not all, causes for headache are:

- Migraine.
- Muscle contraction or tension.
- Infection/inflammation.
- Structural headaches.
- Rebound headaches.

Migraine headaches are caused by some kind of irritation/stimulus in the brain that affects the blood vessels in that part of the brain. These vessels first get small (spasm) and then swell (dilate), causing a throbbing "sick" headache with nausea, vomiting, eye pain with bright lights, and even warning symptoms like shooting lights in the eyes before a headache begins. The headache may last minutes to hours. Migraines can be triggered by stress, foods, smells, or exercise. These headaches tend to run in families.

There are medications that can stop a headache, such as sumatriptan (Imitrex®), and also medications, such as beta-blockers or calcium channel blocker, that can prevent migraines if they are happening frequently.

Migraines can be caused, or worsened, by the use of birth control pills. Any new headaches that occur after beginning birth control pills should be discussed with your doctor.

Infections can also be associated with headaches. Sinus infections generally cause pain in the cheek and forehead area, as well as behind the eyes. Ear infections will hurt in the ears, or sometimes in the area behind or in front of the ears. Meningitis or encephalitis, two life-threatening infections in the fluid around the brain, can also cause severe headaches, usually associated with a stiff neck, fever, rash, and mental confusion.

Bacteria, fungi, or viruses, including the newly recognized West Nile virus, can cause these infections. HIV or other diseases that interfere with your body's ability to fight off germs may invite painful brain infections.

Structural causes for headache include brain tumors and leakage of blood into the brain. These leakages can occur with an aneurysm (weakened area of blood vessel), with subdural hematoma (bleeding that puts pressure on the brain, usually after an injury), and with hemorrhage (bleeding into the brain tissue or into the fluid around the brain). Concussion (bruising of the brain after an injury) is frequently associated with headaches that may last for days or weeks after the injury.

The headaches are often, but not always, associated with other symptoms. Other symptoms may include:

- Nausea and vomiting.
- Localized weakness.
- Changes in vision (actual double vision).
- Worsening of the headache when you cough or sneeze.
- Head pain that awakens you from sleep.

All headaches with a structural origin are very serious and require urgent evaluation and treatment by your doctor or in a hospital emergency room.

Rebound headaches are the kind of headaches you may experience if you stop taking a prescription or over-the-counter pain medicine that you've been using regularly. Rebound headaches can be very difficult to treat. Use of additional pain medications just keeps the rebound cycle going.

For more information see the National Headache Foundation web site at *www.headaches.org*.

ABDOMINAL AND PELVIC PAIN

Pain can occur in any of the organs in the abdomen or pelvis. The stomach and the first part of the intestine (the duodenum) may develop ulcers related to acid, alcohol intake, or an infection caused by the germ *Helicobacter pylori* (*H. pylori*). The pancreas may become inflamed by stones or alcohol intake, or occasionally, without any obvious cause. This inflammation is accompanied by severe pain in the middle upper abdomen. This condition is called "pancreatitis."

The large intestine, or colon, can have pain related to infection, spasm, or blockage. Infections can be widespread–for example, food poisoning caused by bacteria in improperly cooked or stored foods. These infections may also be local to the affected person, such as when a pocket of infection develops in a pouch in the wall of the colon, called "diverticulitis."

Inflammatory bowel disease, or *Crohn's disease*, and ulcerative colitis may cause pain due to spasm and cramping. *Irritable bowel syndrome*, a very common condition affecting both sexes (but women more frequently than men), is associated with changes in bowel function—sometimes diarrhea, sometimes constipation, sometimes alternating diarrhea and constipation in the same person. There is often cramping abdominal pain with this condition.

Gallbladder pain is associated with infection and stones, and is addressed in another section of this chapter. Cancer in any of these organs may also first show itself by pain.

Pelvic pain in women can result from uterus, tube, ovary, cervix, or vagina problems. Infections in any of these organs may result in significant pain, and the infections may also cause infertility.

Cysts in the ovary cause the stretching type of pain. When such a cyst breaks, its fluid leaks into the pelvic cavity, and this causes pain as well.

Complications of pregnancy, including a tubal, or ectopic pregnancy, may first show up with a doctor's visit for pelvic pain or bleeding.

Fibroids (non-cancerous tumors of the uterus) can cause pain, as well as abnormal bleeding.

Pain or cramping that come with the menstrual period, called "dysmenorrhea," is usually well-managed with anti-inflammatory medications. If these don't work, birth control pills can often prevent dysmenorrhea.

Another cause of pelvic pain, especially in women, is a condition called *interstitial cystitis*. A person with this condition feels the need to urinate often, and will experience pain or pressure, including a burning feeling in the pelvic area.

Because examination of the urine shows no signs of infection in these cases, a urologist will often be needed to make sure there are no other bladder diseases present. Medications can be helpful in managing the symptoms of this condition.

Pelvic pain in men can be caused by infections in the bladder or prostate.

Kidney stones may be present with abdominal, pelvic or groin/scrotal pain, and will be discussed more in a later section.

For more information see the International Pelvic Pain Society at *www.pelvicpain.org*.

CANCER

There are many types of cancer specific to the organ or area in the body where the cancer began. Some may start in one place or organ, and then migrate to and attack other parts of the body. The invasion of the cancer cells damages nerves and tissue, and pain results. Pain can also result from the swelling and stretching of the involved organ. Not only the organs but also the bones can be involved. The cells of prostate cancer and breast cancer can travel to the bones and cause bone destruction and daily deep-bone pain.

The most effective way to reduce the pain is to reduce the size and spread of the cancer by means of medications, radiation, or surgery. Pain medications usually begin with the mildest, and then get stronger. A cancer expert (Oncologist) will help coordinate cancer treatment and pain treatment.

Some cancers are untreatable and people die of them. In such cases, hospice services are available for pain control and end-of-life care.

For more information see the American Cancer Society at *www.cancer.org* or the excellent teaching site, *www.Cancerquest.org*.

For hospice information, see chapter 14, The Future of Pain Treatment.

FIBROMYALGIA

Fibromyalgia is a painful condition that affects women more often than men. The symptoms are:

- Sore muscles.
- Aching tissues.
- Sleeping trouble.
- Tiredness.
- Irritable bowel problems (diarrhea, constipation, cramping, or a combination of these).

The presence of "trigger points"—sore spots on the body that cause pain when pressed—is a sign of fibromyalgia. There is usually no abnormal blood test or other clinical findings.

Your primary care doctor, sometimes with the help of a rheumatologist, can best evaluate this condition. First-line pain treatment helps relieve fibromyalgia. Stretching exercises and antidepressants, even when there is no depression, are often effective.

For more information see the Arthritis Foundation web site at *www.arthritis.org*, and the National Institute of Arthritis and Muculoskeletal and Skin Diseases (NIAMS) web site at *www.niams.nih.gov/hi/topics/fibromyalgia.fibrogs.htm*.

INFECTIONS

Infections may cause pain in the infected body part. Kidney infections cause back pain, pneumonia can cause chest pain, and infections in the spinal fluid can cause headaches. Infection in the bone (*osteomyelitis*) can cause localized deep-bone pain.

Having a fever may be a clue that an infection is at work. Visit your doctor and expect to have your blood work checked for a high white blood cell count, and an X-ray or scan of the painful area. Once the infection is identified, your doctor will usually order antibiotics. Pain medication may be necessary while the infection is being treated.

Varicella or *chicken pox* is a childhood virus infection. Once the infection appears to have cleared, the virus can live quietly in the nerve root for many years, and then, without warning, cause a painful attack on the nerve and on the skin supplied by that nerve. When that occurs, the condition that results is called "herpes zoster" or "shingles."

The first sign of shingles is a tingling pain, usually on one side of the body. Skin irritation, redness, and then small blisters appear and may last for a week. This can be treated with antiviral medications like acyclovir and famciclovir, which may shorten the duration and lessen the symptoms.

You are contagious when the blisters appear, and you should stay away from people who have not had chicken pox or who do not have a fully working immune system. You should be treated with Valtrex®, famciclovir, or Zovirax® (acyclovir).

Your doctor should look for a reason why the chicken pox virus reactivated, although usually no cause is found. We do know that you become more vulnerable to shingles as you get older or if your immune system has been weakened. Pain medication on the skin, such as capsaicin (Zostrix®), Xylocaine®, or lidocaine topical or transdermal Lidoderm®, may help.

Another sexually transmitted viral infection that causes pain and small blisters in the genital area is *herpes*. Once you have been infected, you may have repeated reoccurrences. This infection can be passed to your sex partner. The symptoms can be treated with the antiviral medications acyclovir (Zovirax®) or famciclovir.

Pain Matters

Many diseases and conditions that cause pain can be treated with medications that prevent or treat the pain.

STONES

Gallstones and kidney stones are two common causes of pain, produced as the body tries to pass these hard particles through the drainage tubing system.

Gallstones form in several situations. One setting is that life-long breakdown of red blood cells (hemolysis) can cause too much bilirubin to be produced. This can happen to children and teenagers with sickle cell disease or thalassemia. The more common cause, too much cholesterol, is frequently seen in the fourth or fifth decade of life.

Gallstones form in the gall bladder, which sits under the liver in the right upper abdomen. Gallstones cause pain when the gall bladder tries to force them out after one eats a fatty meal. The problem can be fixed by surgical removal of the gall bladder, or, sometimes, by medication to dissolve the stones. Your primary care doctor or an intestinal disease specialist (gastroenterologist) can make the diagnosis, and a general surgeon will help in the treatment.

Kidney stones form when the body releases too much crystal, which gathers in the urine. These crystals form stones, and can become stuck in the ureter, the tube that carries urine from the kidney to the bladder. As the stone is being passed, it can cause intense pain in the back or abdominal region, or in the groin and scrotum.

Treatment includes breaking the stones with sound waves, a procedure called lithotripsy, or by using a catheter to go in through the bladder to pull the stone out, as well as diet changes to prevent crystal formation. A urologist is the best one to manage these stones.

For more information see *www.niddk.nih.gov/health/kidney/pubs/stonadul/stonadul.htm.*

CHAPTER 5

Dealing with the Medical World

Many people are frightened by the medical world because they don't know how it works. Such fear can mean trouble finding the right caregiver, understanding your ailment and its treatment, or even getting the yearly medical checkups and good health tips you need in order to stay healthy. Because pain involves a wide variety of doctors, depending on the source of the pain, you need a scorecard that helps you identify the players. You also need to know how to choose the right doctor for your particular problem. In this chapter, we lay that out for you, and explain what you need to know about pain clinics and about the various insurance programs that can help you with the bills.

WHO'S WHO

MD—Physicians

When dealing with pain, it is good to have a doctor who knows all about you and can coordinate your care. Specialists may only focus on one problem, but a primary care doctor can keep an eye on the big picture.

Who you see may depend on your insurance plan. Usually insurance companies will give you a list of primary-care physicians within the plan from whom you can choose. You can find out a lot about the best available doctors from friends, family, church members, and co-workers. Ask them about whether they are satisfied with the doctor they see. Eventually, this will help you find the right match for yourself.

If the person in pain is a child, your best bet as a coordinator is a *pediatrician,* who specializes in children's health. Doctors who practice *internal medicine* are experts who coordinate care for adults. Family practitioners can coordinate care for both children and adults.

Specialists who help diagnose and treat specific causes of pain are:

Obstetricians and gynecologists (Ob-Gyn) care for women and manage pregnancy, and are also experts in breast and uterine fibroids and in female cancers.

Oncologists are specialists in cancer and cancer-related pain.

Hematologists treat such blood diseases as sickle cell and hemophilia.

Rheumatologists are experts in arthritis and joint problems who are specially trained to manage immune arthritis. They may do joint injections but they do not do surgery.

Podiatrists are experts in all aspects of foot pain and foot surgery. They may overlap with Orthopedic Surgeons.

Radiologists read X-rays and scans to help diagnose problems.

Surgeons operate to correct problems that may be causing pain.

Urologists are experts in the urinary system, including kidney stones.

Orthopedic surgeons are bone specialists who can operate and replace joints damaged by osteoarthritis. Some orthopedic surgeons do back surgery for slipped discs.

Neurologists specialize in migraine, other headaches, and neuropathic pain caused by diabetes and other nerve injuries.

Neurosurgeons operate on brain tumors, slipped discs, and spinal-cord problems.

Emergency medicine doctors staff emergency rooms and are skilled to handle emergency situations.

Anesthesia and pain specialists provide pain management and anesthesia for surgery. They treat prolonged pain that will not go away through the use of pain blocks and pain pumps.

Other experts who can provide treatment for pain are:

Doctor of Osteopathy (DO)

Doctors of Osteopathy, or DOs, have all of the usual medical school training and specialization, plus additional training in bone and muscle manipulation and massage. In most states in the United States, DO licenses are interchangeable with MD licenses, and the practitioners have a similar scope of responsibilities.

Doctor of Chiropractic (DC)

Doctors of Chiropractic or Chiropractors have been trained in spine manipulation to relieve pressure on the nerves in the spinal cord. They may also diagnose the cause of pain related to arthritis using X-rays, and they can help ease pain caused by muscle strain injury.

Physician Assistants (PAs) and Nurse Practitioners (NPs)

Physician Assistants (PAs) and Nurse Practitioners (NPs) are trained to do 90 percent of what doctors do and are supervised by doctors. They have special training in patient education, and will spend time answering questions, doing the medical checkups, seeing patients in the hospital, and coordinating care. PAs and NPs help the doctor to see more patients by spending time with you to handle routine care, and give you information.

Nurses

Nurses are the educators, medication providers, care coordinators, and counselors to patients and their family members. While you are in the hospital, nurses are responsible for 24-hour delivery of medications, monitoring of your condition, and tracking your vital signs along with your pain and fluid levels. Nurses can be specialized (as for example, pain management experts or experts in critical care), or they can be generalists. Some nurses can administer antibiotics and pain medication in your home, if home visit programs are available in your community.

Psychiatrists and Psychologists

Psychiatrists are medical doctors with special training in psychiatry and the use of medications to help depression, anxiety, and emotional disorders. Psychologists are trained to provide counseling, testing, and emotional support for the same issues. Chronic pain may precipitate emotional stresses that need help from professionals.

Both psychiatrists and psychologists can teach patients how to use biofeedback, distraction, and relaxation techniques to help control pain.

Social Workers

Social workers are experts in helping you solve such social issues as insurance coverage, job and school issues, housing problems, and medical disability. They also help arrange hospice and home-health services, do crisis counseling, and help families get back on their feet after setbacks. Social workers are usually employed by hospitals, sickle cell centers, and health departments. Some states have vocational rehabilitation services that provide skill testing, job readiness, and job-training programs. The clinic or hospital social worker should be the most knowledgeable about these programs in your state.

Chaplains

Chaplains are ministers employed by hospitals and clinics to help meet the spiritual needs of patients in the hospital. A healthy spiritual life helps you to maintain hope and a positive outlook. The leader at your local house of worship can play an important role on your health care team by helping you work out issues of guilt, depression, fear (such as fear of death), and hopelessness.

Physical Therapists

Physical therapists are trained to help exercise and strengthen muscles and joints after surgery or injury. They are experts in using heat, cold, massages, and exercise to help mend injured muscles and joints. They help train patients to use transcutaneous nerve stimulation (TNS) to block chronic pain. They can help you through rehabilitation and show you different ways to get through daily life when the usual ways do not work or cause pain. Physical therapists are found in hospitals, pain clinics, orthopedic clinics, home health agencies, and freestanding therapy centers.

Vocational Rehabilitation

Vocational Rehabilitation experts are trained to help you get job training and retraining. They try to match patients with jobs that will not add new medical problems to the chronic conditions they already have. If your job is causing problems, this is the expert you want to see. Vocational rehabilitators are usually employed by the state government or by rehabilitation programs. Your social worker can help you contact these services.

FINDING THE RIGHT HEALTH CARE PROVIDER

To find a healthcare provider to help manage your pain or any other health issues, start with a primary-care provider. For adults, this is an internal medicine provider or family practitioner. If you can't get good leads from family, friends, etc., call your local medical society or hospital for a referral to a primary-care provider.

The qualities you will want in a provider are:

- Willingness to take the time to listen to your issues and to explain your diagnosis and treatment options.
- Willingness to take your pain seriously and believe your level of pain.
- Willingness to partner with you to help you overcome the pain.

Contact your state's medical board to make sure the provider is certified, and not under investigation by the board. Contact information is usually in the phone book, but if you don't find it, ask your local librarian to help. If you need a specialist, your primary-care provider should be able to recommend and refer you to the best one.

Your provider may want you to sign a pain treatment contract. In such a contract, the provider promises to provide you the best possible pain management, and you promise to use only pain medications the provider prescribes, to follow the treatment plans, and not to sell your pain medications. Such a contract is a good, practical step in a long-term partnership.

PAIN CLINICS

Your family doctor, internist, or, for your children, a pediatrician can help you find a pain clinic. If you have HMO insurance, you may have an assigned primary care giver and clinic. The clinician may be excellent, or may have very little pain management experience. In the latter case, ask the clinician for referral to a specialist or pain expert near your home. This may require an appeal through your health plan, asking for the best pain care available in your community.

Pain clinics are relatively new to the medical world. They are usually run by physicians who are pain experts. These experts tend to be anesthesiologists or neurologists experienced in treating long lasting and difficult pain. Pain clinics may offer comprehensive services, including physical therapy, pain counselors, pain blocks (with which numbing medication is injected in the painful areas), and surgical procedures.

Pain specialists are usually members of two professional organizations: the American Pain Society (*www.ampainsoc.org*), or the American Board of Pain Medicine (*www.abpm.org*). Look for physicians in your area who are members of one of these groups.

EMERGENCY ROOMS

If you are suffering intense pain at 2 A.M., you are usually dependent on the local emergency room for pain management. Unfortunately, the ER is usually the place where there is the most resistance to using pain medication, the highest suspicion that you are drug-seeking, and the most unbelievable about your pain level.

That's why, especially in the ER, you must be proactive. Being proactive means:

- Doing research *before* you need the emergency room, so that you know in advance who in your community would serve you best in pain management.

- Getting recommendations from your regular doctor, other patients, families, and pain associations and centers.
- Having your regular health care provider write up an emergency room plan that includes your medical history, physical findings, lab values, and medications to use for pain. Have this plan placed in a notebook in the emergency room or in your hospital. Also keep one copy to take with you to show the nurses and physicians in the ER.

> *Especially in the ER, you must be proactive.*

In dealing with the staff of the ER, you have to be proactive and know what you need for proper treatment. Identify nurses and physicians in the ER who are champions for pain management and who can make sure you get proper treatment.

THE SPECIALIST

Your family or emergency room doctor may refer you to a specialist to manage your pain. Migraine headaches may need the evaluation of a Neurologist; rheumatoid arthritis may need the care of a Rheumatologist; and cancer is best managed by an Oncologist.

But even while you are working with a specialist, keep seeing your family doctor, who understands the big picture. Some specialists do become your primary-care doctor, but this is rare and you should not depend on it.

COST OF CARE

The most expensive cost you will have is the hospital charges for inpatient stays. The average hospital stay for pain treatment is five days, with an average cost of $6500, though costs vary from city to city and hospital to hospital. That's one of many reasons why prevention can be more important than finding a cure. It reduces the need to stay in the hospital and reduces costs dramatically.

Visits to the local emergency room will cost anywhere from $200 to $1000 per visit and regular checkups with your healthcare provider cost about $200 per visit. Your insurance program may help cover the costs of such visits.

Cost for tests and lab work can add to the bill. The most expensive test is the MRI, which runs more than $1,500. The most expensive treatments are surgery, and therapy that uses nerve blocks or pain pumps. Work with your doctor, insurance company, and social worker to work out the most cost-effective plan.

Medications for pain, especially the new COX-2 NSAIDs, are very expensive. Many drug companies have patient support programs that help you get the medication you need at prices you can afford. These programs usually require paperwork, filled out by your doctor, that demonstrates need.

Medication is usually provided one month at a time. Ordering your medication from mail order companies can save money. Shop around for the best deal. There are mail order companies in Canada that ship medication to the U.S. at reduced prices.

Social workers, who are experts in resources and state governmental rules, can help you to cut down out-of-pocket costs. Usually social workers are based at the local hospital in your community.

INSURANCE PLANS: HMOS, PPOS, MEDICARE AND MEDICAID

HMOs

Traditional "fee-for-service" insurance plans allow you to see any doctor you want. After you have met an annual deductible (which varies from one plan to another), the plan will pay the doctor or hospital 70–85 percent of the approved amount for the doctor's services, depending on your plan. Fee for service health plans are usually the most expensive kind of healthcare insurance, but they offer the most freedom of choice.

HMO is the common term for health maintenance organizations that provide managed care plans. Depending on your plan, you either pick or are assigned to a primary care provider, or PCP, from an approved list. This provider may be a family practitioner, a pediatrician, an internist, a gynecologist, a geriatrician (a specialist in the care of older adults), a physician assistant, or a nurse practitioner.

The PCP is in charge of your overall care and acts as the gatekeeper for all of your healthcare, deciding what tests you will have done and which specialists you will need.

HMO's usually do a good job of preventive care because preventing complications saves them money. They are good at managing people who are generally healthy, but chronic disease can be a challenge to this system. You may start to run into resistance from your HMO on issues of treatment and referral to pain specialists. Your PCP may choose a less expensive treatment, even though it might not be the most effective or have the fewest side effects.

Some HMO's might still deny payment for more aggressive treatments for chronic pain, such as pain pumps, pain blocks, or comprehensive pain management. If you are denied treatment or service you think you are entitled to, remember that HMO's have an appeals process. Start with your PCP and work up the chain of command. Some states have insurance advocate offices to which you can appeal.

PPOs

PPOs, or preferred provider organizations, are another large category of health care providers. In this type of plan you may or may not have a PCP as gatekeeper. Often, you can simply see any specialist who participates in the plan, without referral from a PCP.

Some PPOs pay a portion of fees for visits to doctors outside their network, although in such a case you will be responsible for a larger portion of the fee than if you saw a doctor within the network.

Medicare and Medicaid

The Federal government runs two kinds of healthcare plans. *Medicaid* is government insurance available to indigent people in all states and territories of the United States, as well as Puerto Rico and Washington, D.C. The specific requirements that an individual or family must meet to qualify for Medicaid vary from state to state. The best source of information on your state's requirements is a social worker or the local Medicaid office.

For more information, see *www.cms.hhs.gov/medicaid/*.

Medicare is government insurance for people 65 years of age and older. Disabled people under 65 can apply for Medicare coverage, as can people with End-Stage Renal Disease (permanent kidney failure treated with dialysis or a transplant).

Medicare has two parts:

Part A—Hospital Insurance: Most people do not have to pay for Part A. It covers:

- Care in hospitals as an inpatient.
- Critical access hospitals (small facilities that give limited outpatient and inpatient services to people in rural areas).
- Skilled nursing facilities.
- Hospice care.
- Some home healthcare.

Part B—Medical Insurance: Most people pay monthly for Part B of Medicare. It covers doctors' services, outpatient hospital care, and some other medical services that Part A does not cover, such as the services of physical and occupational therapists, and some home healthcare. Part B helps pay for these covered services and supplies when they are medically necessary.

For more information see *www.medicare.gov.*

Another Social Security program for the disabled is *SSI.* To be awarded SSI, a person has to fulfill the same requirements as for Social Security Disability, except that the applicant need never have worked. SSI is a Federal income supplement program funded by general tax revenues (*not* Social Security taxes).

SSI is designed to help aged, blind, and disabled people who have little or no income. It provides these people cash to meet their basic needs: food, clothing, and shelter. The financial award provided by SSI is usually less than what one receives with a disability award. SSI does *not* lead to Medicare coverage.

For more information see *www.ssa.gov/disability.*

Pain Matters

In this chapter you have learned how to navigate the medical world to get the best possible treatment for your pain. Treatment may require that you be involved with several members of the healthcare team, and knowing their roles will help you know what to expect, and what to do if your pain is not getting better. You have also learned the kinds of insurance programs that can help you pay your medical bills.

CHAPTER 6

Assessing Pain

FINDING THE CAUSE

When you first visit your Primary Care Provider (PCP), there's a clear agenda—to pin down the area of the pain, and, if possible, to find its cause. Coming up with the right answers can sometimes be easy—for example, if the trouble started when you lifted a heavy box without bending your knees and felt a pop in your lower back, followed by intense pain. But pinning down the cause can be far more complicated. For many people, pain doesn't come in all at once. Instead, pain creeps in. A nuisance at first, it only gradually builds up to a serious problem. Such pain may even move around, making the cause even harder to find.

YOUR MEDICAL HISTORY—TELL THE STORY!

Did you know that 70 percent of your diagnosis comes from your descriptions of the pain? Don't make the doctor drag those details out of you. Be ready to describe your pain, as exactly as possible. It's helpful to write down your description of the pain before the actual visit, so that when you get to the doctor's office you know what you want to tell him or her. Here's a little memory aid to help you with your description. It's called LOCATES.

L—*Location.* Exactly where is the pain coming from and does it travel to other parts? For example, classic sciatica back pain from a slipped disc may hurt in the lower back, but sciatica also sends shooting pains that travel down the backs of your legs.

O—*Other associated symptoms* that have occurred along with the pain—such as nausea, vomiting, a stiff neck, sweating, shortness of breath, and so forth.

C—*Character of the pain.* Just what does the pain feel like to you? Is it throbbing, constant, sharp, dull, shooting, stabbing, burning, or any other word that helps describe your pain?

A—*Alleviating or Aggravating circumstances.* What makes the pain better? Have your tried heat, ice, rest, or any pain medications? What makes the pain worse: exertion, movement, deep breathing, eating, bending, or anything else?

T—*Timing.* When did the pain start? Has it been constant or does it come and go? How long have you had the pain? Is it brand-new or an old guest who won't leave?

E—*Environment.* Where were you and what were you doing at the time the pain started? Do you have the pain only at work or only when you lie flat, or only when you walk up a hill, etc.?

S—*Severity.* How would you rate the pain at its worst moment? How would you rate it at present? Use a scale of 0–10, where zero is no pain and 10 is the worst pain you've ever had.

Take a few minutes right now to write down your individual LOCATES.

Once you've told your doctor how you experience the pain, he or she will ask you about your past medical history, including:

- Allergies.
- Past hospitalizations.
- Major illnesses (like diabetes, heart disease, kidney problems, etc.).
- Surgeries.
- Injuries.
- Medications, including health food supplements and vitamins.

Your PCP should also ask you if anyone in your family has similar pain problems. (If the PCP forgets to ask, remind him or her.) Information about your family's health histories helps identify genetic causes.

Finally, your PCP will explore your social history, as it might be pertinent to your health. Expect questions about your family life, food intake, lifestyle, smoking, alcohol use, street-drug use, personal relationships, employment, and support systems—including home life, friends, family, and religion. These can all give clues to the cause of your pain, and help the PCP come up with possible treatment options that will work best for you.

THE PHYSICAL EXAMINATION

The PCP should examine you by taking your temperature and blood pressure, and by looking at the areas surrounding the pain. The physical examination should include a thorough examination of the area that is causing the pain. Because pain can travel from its origin to other body locations, the PCP may examine several body parts while searching for clues to the cause.

LAB WORK

The location of the pain and the probable causes will direct which blood tests, if any, may be helpful to the diagnosis. Pain cannot be measured by blood tests, but in certain situations blood tests may help pinpoint the cause of pain. For example, the cause of chest pain can be investigated with blood tests that show whether the patient has had a heart attack. By the same token, if an infection is suspected as the cause of the pain, your doctor might order a complete blood count and take cultures.

There are blood tests that can measure inflammation in the body. If the tests are elevated, there is usually inflammation in the body caused by the body's attacking itself, an invading infection, or a tumor.

CT, MRI, THERMOGRAPHY

If your doctor suspects that the cause of the pain may be arthritis, a bone tumor, or a fracture, he or she may order special films to help diagnose the source of the pain. Getting pictures with the help of CAT scan and MRI lets the doctor see into organs, tissues, and bones. These tests can help discover pinched nerves, tumors, or blockages in an organ.

The clinician may also order more specialized scans, such as bone scans, to check for bone infections or tumors that may not show up using the other methods.

Thermography identifies areas in the body where there is increased heat from increased blood flow. Thermography can help identify areas where inflammation is occurring. Because thermography is not available everywhere, many healthcare providers do not use it to diagnose pain.

PAIN BY LOCATION: HEAD, NECK, CHEST, BELLY, BACK, JOINTS

The specific location of the pain in the body can be an important clue as to causes. Possible locations are listed below.

Head Pain

Meningitis is an infection in the spinal fluid that surrounds your brain and spinal cord. It can cause fever, headache, nausea, vomiting, eye pain in bright lights, neck stiffness, skin rash, and confusion. If you experience these symptoms in some combination, you need medical evaluation immediately.

Migraine headaches are caused by blood vessels in the brain first shrinking and then swelling, causing a one-sided, throbbing, "sick" headache, with nausea, vomiting, eye pain in bright lights, and even warning symptoms in the form of shooting lights in the eyes before a headache begins.

Migraine headaches, which are thought to be inherited, can be triggered by stress, foods, smells, or exercise. The headache may last minutes or hours. Medications such as sumatriptan (Imitrex®) can stop a headache. Others, such as beta-blockers or calcium channel-blockers, can help prevent frequent migraines.

Tension or stress headaches can be caused by stress and worry, but also by posture, neck problems, or other causes of muscle tightness. When muscles in the neck and scalp become tense, tension pain may feel like a tight band around the head going into the neck, or around the neck where it meets the head. The pain is treated with heat, massage, stress reduction, and first-level pain treatment. In long-lasting cases, preventative medications may need to be used on a daily basis to prevent the headache, rather than waiting for it to begin, and then treating it.

Sinus infections cause pain in the front of the head above the eyes, or deep between the eyes where your sinuses are located. Infected sinuses swell and throb.

Treatment includes antibiotic medication, decongestants, and first-level pain treatment.

Eye problems include increased eye pressure, or glaucoma, as well as eyestrain, both of which can cause headache. There are medications to lower the eye pressure if this is the cause.

Brain tumor or abscess. Any swelling in the brain can cause a severe headache. The swelling may also cause nausea, vomiting, blurred vision, and weakness. Brain tumor or abscess can be diagnosed through the use of a MRI or CT scan.

Neck pain

Neck arthritis, as well as a slipped disc, causes neck pain that is made worse by movement. The patient may feel tingling in the arm and/or hand, along with a feeling of weakness. X-rays of the neck, and a CT or MRI may help make the diagnosis. Treatment with first-level pain treatments, as well as physical therapy, is best. In some extreme cases, surgery may be needed.

Stress can cause the large muscles in the back of the neck to contract and cause pain. Treatment includes first-level pain management, heat, massage, and stress reduction.

Referred pain from the heart. Angina (pain from an oxygen-starved heart) can cause the neck to hurt. This pain is usually on the left side of the neck and is brought on by exercise or stress.

Chest Pain

Angina is a feeling of chest heaviness or tightness, or a feeling of squeezing pain in the chest, neck, and left arm. Angina is often brought on by heavy exertion or stress. It is caused by blocked blood flow in the main blood vessels that supply oxygen to the heart muscle pumping your blood. Angina is a warning sign that a complete blockage may occur, causing a heart attack. If you experience any of these symptoms, get to the emergency room immediately, and have someone inform your PCP.

Treatment includes a daily baby aspirin to prevent blood clotting, and nitroglycerine tablets to use if the chest pain recurs. A visit to the cardiologist, or heart specialist, will be arranged for special tests to see if the blockage can be fixed.

Abdominal causes such as gallstones, ulcers, and esophagitis can cause pain in the chest.

Lung causes, such as pneumonia, collapsed lung, or blood clots in the lung, can also be associated with pain, along with shortness of breath that's made worse when you take a deep breath. This is a serious symptom and you need to be evaluated immediately in an emergency room.

Chest pain can also be caused by *heart valve problems* that slow the blood flow through the heart and lungs. Valve problems can be diagnosed by echocardiogram (a special heart ultrasound test) and a consultation with a cardiologist (heart expert).

Pericarditis, an infection of the sack that surrounds the heart, can be diagnosed by EKG and echocardiogram.

Shingles (Herpes Zoster) can cause intense skin pain in a line from the back to the chest, followed by a rash of clear small blisters. Shingles is caused by the same virus that causes chicken pox. The virus can live quietly in the nerves for many years, and then appear with pain and rash during times of stress or for no reason at all. Shingles is treated early with the antiviral medications acyclovir (Zovirax®) or famciclovir (Famvir®) when the first symptoms occur, to speed recovery.

Belly Pain

Ulcers can be caused by infection in the stomach or by pain medications in the aspirin and NSAID family (see Chapter 8). Treatment includes antibiotics and acid blockers.

Gallstones form when there is too much bilirubin produced, as a result of a lifetime of red blood cells breaking apart. Such breaking apart of cells can happen to children and teenagers with sickle cell disease or thalassemia. More commonly, gallstones, caused by cholesterol, are seen in people in their 40s or 50s.

Gallstones form in the gall bladder, which sits under the liver in the right upper abdomen. The stones cause pain when the gall bladder tries to force them out after one eats a fatty meal.

The problem can be fixed by removing the gall bladder with the stones by surgery, or by medication to dissolve the stones. A Gastroenterologist and, sometimes, a general surgeon best manage treatment of gallstones.

Appendicitis causes pain that can start in the belly button area and settle in the lower right abdomen. It can cause fever, nausea, vomiting, and loss of appetite. Surgery to remove the appendix is the best therapy.

In females, belly pain can be related to:

- Menstrual cycle.
- Ovarian cysts.
- Fibroids.
- Ovulation.
- Ectopic pregnancy.
- Pelvic infections.
- Bladder infections.

All abdominal pain should be evaluated by a heathcare provider as quickly as possible.

Back Pain

Back strain occurs when a back muscle is stretched or strained by lifting or injury. There are no abnormal X-rays or blood tests that diagnose back strain.

First-line pain therapy with NSAIDs, physical therapy, and special back exercises are the best treatments. Bed rest does not work. The best way to recover is by staying active and returning to normal activities as much as the pain allows.

Kidney stones form when the body releases too much of a chemical that produces crystals in the urine. These stones can become stuck in the ureter, the tube that carries urine from the kidney to the bladder. Kidney stones can cause intense back pain as they are being passed.

Treatment includes breaking the stones with sound waves called "lithotripsy," using a catheter to go in through the bladder to pull the stone out, and making diet changes to prevent crystal formation. A Urologist is a doctor specially trained to manage these stones.

Kidney infection is caused by bacteria that first infect the urine tubing, and then enter the kidney. The infection can cause back pain, fever, nausea, and vomiting. It is treated with antibiotics and first line pain therapy.

Slipped disc. The disc is a jelly-like pad that separates the vertebrae that make up the backbone. A disc can bulge out of position. This bulge, caused by pushing on the nerves coming out of the spinal cord, causes pain and possibly weakness along the area supplied by the nerve. A slipped disc is diagnosed by MRI.

First-line pain therapy and limited activity is the initial treatment. Surgery may be needed if the irritation continues.

Tumors and infections. Certain cancers, especially prostate and breast, can travel to the bones in the back and cause pain. Multiple Myeloma, a rarer cancer, also causes bone pain. Infections such as tuberculosis and bacteria can infect the bones in the back. Treatments will vary, and are best managed by specialists.

Spinal stenosis is a narrowing of the canal that holds the spinal cord and can cause back pain, pain in both legs, weakness and numbness. Again, treatment varies from case to case, and should be managed by specialists.

Joint Pain

Fast swelling, pain, heat, or redness in one joint is a medical emergency, and could indicate a joint infection. Usually, your physician will drain the joint fluid and have it tested for infection, crystals, and other causes.

Long-term swelling and pain in the fingers, shoulders, knees, and elbows may be caused by osteoarthritis, or simply by the wear and tear on the joint over time. This may show up on X-rays. First-line pain therapy is the best plan.

Long-term swelling, heat, or redness in the joints may be from the body attacking itself or from autoimmune arthritis. This condition includes rheumatoid arthritis, psoriasis, sarcoidosis, systemic lupus erythematosis, and ulcerative bowel disease. Blood tests and X-rays may help confirm the diagnosis. In addition to first-line pain therapy, there may be medicines specific to each disease.

Crystals in the joint fluid can cause gout and pseudo-gout. First-line pain therapy is a good starting point.

PUT A NUMBER ON THAT PAIN

Pain is best given a number by you, the person who is experiencing the pain. Most hospitals use a scale from 0 (no pain) to 10 (the worst pain imaginable). Think about where your pain would fall along this 0 to 10 scale. Having a number to describe your pain level helps doctors and nurses to decide what level of pain treatment to use, and it gives everyone a way to see how your treatment is going. Before treatment begins, the doctor or nurse should ask you about your pain level, and then ask again several times during your treatment to check your progress.

By being honest abut your pain level, you gain the right to be believed. Playing games with your health is dangerous because if you overstate your pain, you could be overmedicated.

You should be familiar with the several different pain scales used in hospitals and doctor's offices. You can settle on the scale that best suits you, and make entries daily. Bring it with you for your healthcare visits.

The following are pain scales you're most likely to see in use:

Visual Analog Scale, or VAS

This is a 10 cm (10 centimeters) line, with "no pain" at the left end and "the worst possible pain" at the right end. You mark the number or point on the line that best corresponds with the level of your pain. The heathcare provider will measure how far your mark is from the "no pain" end and record your pain level in centimeters.

0-to-10 Verbal and Picture Scale

This is a variation that includes pictures. The healthcare worker will ask you to rate your pain verbally on the same scale as above, using both numbers and drawings to guide you.

0-to-10 Faces Scale

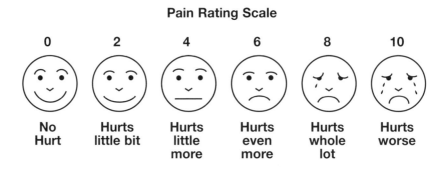

Pain Rating Scale

0	2	4	6	8	10
No Hurt	Hurts little bit	Hurts little more	Hurts even more	Hurts whole lot	Hurts worse

Can't Communicate Scale

Even if you are in pain and can't communicate, your facial expression, posture, and the sounds you make all help the doctor rate your pain level. Based on this same method, there is even a pain scale for babies who can't talk.

These non-verbal scales are usually used in the hospital or nursing home setting.

PAIN IN THREE DIMENSIONS

Pain is multidimensional, and current pain assessment methods such as the visual analog scale and the faces scale only capture one dimension: pain intensity. There is a three-dimensional tool called the "Memorial Pain Card." This tool captures your pain level, your mood level (good or bad), and the amount of your pain relief on three 0-to-10 scales. This scale is not used very often because it requires extra work, even though it provides much more information.

The Memorial Pain Card

1 **Pain Scale**	**2** **Word Description Scale**
Least possible pain ├————————┤ Worst possible pain	Moderate Just noticeable Strong No pain Mild Excruciating Severe Weak
3 **Relief Scale**	**4** **Mood Scale**
No relief of pain ├————————┤ Complete relief of pain	Worst mood ├————————┤ Best mood

Above chart from: Fishman, B, Pasternaks, et. al. The Memorial Pain Assessment Card, *Cancer* 60: 1151–1158, 1987

DOCUMENTING PAIN AND MOOD

People who best help manage their pain keep track of it daily in a pain diary like the one you will find in Appendix A. Write down the date, time, and any treatment you used for the pain. At the time of your visits, share the diary with your doctor or nurse. Your diary can help them know if the pain treatment is working.

You should also decide what pain level you can live with, knowing that being completely free of pain may not be possible. Many people have daily pain scores of 2–3 and are able to do their normal daily routines. How much pain can *you* tolerate and still live a normal life?

In tracking your own pain, watch for mood changes.

The signs of depression are:

- Sleeping too much or too little.
- Having trouble falling asleep.
- Waking up early and not being able to go back to sleep.
- Eating too much or too little.
- Lack of pleasure in things you ordinarily like to do.
- Lack of any fun in life.
- Withdrawal from normal life activities.

Note if you are fearful or anxious about things that didn't bother you before. All of these issues need to be brought to the attention of your doctor, who may recommend medications and treatment that can help.

For more information on pain assessment, see Appendix A.

Pain Matters

With your help, your doctor can find the source of your pain and treat it accordingly. Pain needs to be tracked over time to determine if it is improving under treatment. Tools like pain scales and pain diaries can help you communicate your pain levels to your healthcare team.

Part Two

TREATING PAIN

Dosages and specific medications are only suggestions. The information is not exhaustive and does not cover all ailments, physical conditions, or all their treatments. Only your healthcare provider can know your particular case and design the treatment plan best for you.

CHAPTER 7

An Overview of Pain Treatments

THE ABCS

The ABCs together with the Three Step approach offer a simple way to manage pain. The ABCs are:

A—*Assess* the pain by doing the LOCATES (see Chapter 6).

B—*Believe* the person in pain, whether you are a friend or relative, or the doctor doing the evaluation. Pain cannot be measured from the outside.

C—*Choose* the safest treatment for your pain. Use the World Health Organization (WHO) Three-step Ladder. The first step is for mild pain, a 1 to 3 on the 10–point scale. The second step is for moderate pain, a 4 to 6. The third step is severe pain, a 7 to 10 (See treatments below.)

D—*Deliver* the treatment in the safest manner. Pain medicine should be given at set time intervals, not whenever the pain returns. Taking medication by mouth is usually safer than intravenously or by injection. At the same time, pain medicine may not work as fast when given by mouth because it must first be absorbed by the stomach.

E—*Educate* yourself about the cause and the treatments of your pain. Become an empowered consumer and, by teaching others, an advocate for good pain care.

If the pain is from an acute injury or muscle strain, remember the RICE treatment for the first 24 to 48 hours:

R—*Rest* the injured area.

I—*Ice* the injured area (10 to 20 minutes on and 20 off).

C—*Compress* the area to prevent swelling (Ace bandage wrap).

E—*Elevate* the area to prevent swelling.

After 48 hours, switch from using ice to using heat by heating pad or moist warm towels.

THE THREE-STEP WHO LADDER (FROM THE WORLD HEALTH ORGANIZATION

The World Health Organization's three-step approach to pain treatment is widely accepted by pain experts around the world. (Medication details are available in the next chapter.)

First Level (0-3 Level)—Mild Pain

Medications

Start with one of the following non-opiate medications:

- Acetaminophen.
- Aspirin.
- Ibuprofen.
- Naproxyn.
- Ketoprofen.
- On the skin—capsacin and lidocaine.

Non-medication Treatments

The non-medication treatments for first level pain include:

- Heat: moist heat from a towel soaked in warm water, a warm bath or shower.
- Cold: a cold pack, a pack of frozen peas.
- Massage.
- Relaxation.
- Distraction: watch a movie, listen to your favorite music, do your hobby.
- Rest.

Second level (4–6 level)—Moderate Pain

Medications

Along with first-level pain medications, use mild opiates such as codeine and hydrocodone. Consider the use of antidepressants and, if there is neuropathic pain, seizure medications.

Non-medication Treatments

In addition to all of the treatments in step one, add:

- Acupuncture.
- Physical Therapy.

- Biofeedback.

Third level (7—10 level)—Severe Pain

Medications

The third level involves adding strong opiates such as:

- Morphine.
- Methadone.
- Oxycodone.
- Fentanyl.
- Consider antidepressants.
- Consider seizure medications.

Non-medication Treatments

In addition to levels one and two, consider job rehabilitation if you can no longer do your former work.

Consider becoming part of a clinical trial or research study. People who are in trials and studies do better than those who aren't.

Get a referral to a pain specialist if you aren't working with one already.

Pain Matters

In this chapter, you've learned how to take an organized approach to dealing with your pain, one step at a time.

CHAPTER 8

Non-Opiate Pain Medications

In this chapter we will review the leading non-opiate pain medications available. We will start with pain medications that are applied to the skin. We will then turn to medications that are taken by mouth or by injection. The doses will be listed in milligrams (mg). Doses for children are calculated by the child's weight in kilograms. To convert your child's weight from pounds (lbs) to kilograms (kg), divide it by 2.2. For example: If your child weighs 44 pounds, his/her weight in kilograms would be calculated by dividing 44 by 2.2, which equals 20 kg. If the dose of acetaminophen calls for giving your child 10mg per kg every 4 to 6 hours, you would multiply the weight in kg, or 20, by 10, which equals 200 mg.

We will list the medications by their generic name and then list several of the brand names you may know. An example is the generic medication acetaminophen, whose trade names include Tylenol®, Datril®, and Panadol®. Some medications have too many brand names to list in this book, but all of them should have the same ingredients and the same generic name.

ON THE SKIN

Topical medications, a category of drugs designed to be applied on the skin rather than injected or swallowed, are most commonly used in cases of neuralgia, arthritis, and muscle pain.

Capsaicin

Capsaicin extracts, found naturally in red peppers, are available in two forms: Zostrix® and Zostrix-HP®. Capsaicin has been used for centuries to treat pain.

The first time you apply capsaicin cream to your skin, it will cause redness, swelling, itching, burning, and pain. Soon after you apply the cream, the nerves will become insensitive, and you will no longer feel pain, burning, or itching. To block pain, capsaicin cream must be applied repeatedly and frequently to the painful area.

If you have had permanent nerve damage from shingles, applying capsaicin cream to the area every hour can block the pain. If you have burning or pain in your feet from nerves damaged by diabetes, applying capsaicin cream can block the pain. Exciting new research shows that applying capsaicin cream every hour or two to the skin over painful joints can also block the pain of osteoarthritis, and applying the cream to the nose can prevent cluster headaches and migraines. However, the cream can burn the skin, so stop applying it immediately if you feel continued pain or burning beyond the first application.

Lidocaine

For neuropathic pain, a more useful topical medication, especially for shingles, is the local anesthetic lidocaine. This is the same medicine the dentist uses to numb your mouth and teeth. Available in patch form under the brand name Lidoderm®, the lidocaine patch has the added benefit of protecting the sensitive skin underneath. Lidocaine is also available as a cream or jelly to be applied on the skin over the area with pain.

MEDICATIONS TAKEN BY MOUTH (ORALLY) OR INJECTION

Acetaminophen

Acetaminophen (Tylenol®, Panadol®, and many other brand names) is similar to aspirin in strength, and fever-reducing and pain-reducing ability. The adult dose is 500 mg–1,000 mg by mouth, every four to six hours, for a total not to go over 4,000 mg a day. The dose for children is 10 to 15 mg per kg of body weight by mouth, every four to six hours.

The major difference between acetaminophen and aspirin is that acetaminophen does not cause stomach ulcers, bleeding, blood-clot slowing, or Reye's syndrome. These are all good differences. It does not block inflammation, however, and that may be one reason to choose a medication in the NSAID class.

Acetaminophen can cause liver damage if you go above the 4,000 mg maximum adult daily dose. This risk is increased if you drink more than three alcoholic drinks daily (beer, wine, coolers, etc.).

Salicylate Salts

These pain medications are easier on the stomach than aspirin, and they do not block platelets or slow down the bloodclotting system. The two varieties of this medication are:

- Choline magnesium Trisalicylate (Trilisate®). Dose 1,000 mg—1,500 mg every twelve hours. Maximum dose 3,000 mg a day
- Salsalate (Disalcid®). Dose 1,000 mg—1,500 mg every twelve hours. Maximum dose 3,000 mg a day

Steroids

Steroids are the most potent blockers of inflammation. When osteoarthritis or bursitis is accompanied by inflammation, as indicated by warmth and an accumulation of fluid in the joint, your healthcare provider may recommend that some joint fluid be removed. After fluid is removed, a corticosteroid drug can be injected into the joint. This procedure usually has short-term effects and is used almost exclusively for acute (sudden) and severe symptoms, especially for osteoarthritis of the knee.

Recognize that overuse of this procedure has risks, including an increased risk of infection, thinning of the skin, and tendon rupture. Regular steroid use has some dangers; It can sometimes cause ulcers, loss of calcium, and psychological disturbance. Because of these potential dangers, your health care provider will recommend this treatment only when absolutely necessary.

Steroids are available for use on the skin to block inflammation and itching. They are also available to take by mouth, but only for a short period of time because of unwanted side effects. When you are ready to stop using steroids, they should be reduced gradually.

NON STEROIDAL ANTI-INFLAMMATORY DRUGS—NSAIDS*

All of the medications listed in this category block pain and inflammation (the redness, swelling, and heat in the skin, muscles, and

---

° Advisory: The U.S. Food and Drug Administration (FDA) has issued a public health advisory concerning use of nonsteroidal anti-inflammatory drug products (NSAIDs), including those known as COX-2 selective agents. Recently released data from controlled clinical trials show that the COX-2 selective agents may be associated with an increased risk of serious cardiovascular events (heart attack and stroke) especially when they are used for long periods of time or in very high risk settings (immediately after heart surgery). For more information, please go to the FDA's Web site at *http://www.fda.gov/cder/drug/advisory/nsaids/htm.*

joints). They help ease arthritis, injury, cancer, and menstrual pain. NSAIDs have a maximum dose that should not be exceeded, or serious side effects may occur.

NSAIDs can be purchased without a prescription at reasonable costs. The same medication may be marketed under many different brand names (Bayer®, Anacin®, etc.), but they all have the same ingredients.

Always read the package to see what is in the pill, the strength of the pill in mg, and whether it contains additives. Many NSAIDs also contain other drugs such as caffeine and ingredients for cold medicines.

Unwanted side effects can occur if you mix medications in this category. Pick one and give it a test at the recommended dose. If it doesn't work, stop and switch to a different medication. What works fine for one person may not work for another. Before giving up on this family of medications, keep trying different ones until you find the one that best suits you.

Here is what NSAIDs do:

- Lower fever.
- Block platelets and slows blood clotting. You should not take these medications if you have a problem with excessive bleeding and bruising. Tell your doctor or dentist about the problem before having surgery or any procedure that may cause bleeding. The doctor may have you stop using the NSAID several days before the procedure to make sure you will not bleed too much.
- May cause stomach upset and can cause bleeding ulcers. This problem can be reduced by taking medication to protect your stomach lining (misoprostal 100–200 mcg twice a day, omeprazole 20 mg once daily, or one of the new classes of NSAIDs called COX-2 inhibitors). Stomach problems related to NSAIDs are worse if you drink over three alcoholic beverages daily.

- May damage kidneys, causing foot swelling, and raise blood pressure. Talk to your doctor first before taking these medications if you have kidney problems, heart failure, or high blood pressure.
- Ceiling Effect. The ceiling effect is that there is a point at which taking more of the medicine will not give you more pain relief, but *will* give you more unwanted side effects. This ceiling dose is the maximum amount listed for each medication. If you reach the ceiling dose and still have pain, another medication from a different family of medication, like opiates, should be added.
- NSAIDs can cause headaches as well as treat them.

NSAIDs present no tolerance problems, physical or psychological dependence, or risk of addiction.

NSAIDs cannot be taken together with medicines in the same family. For example, you should not take Ibuprofen (Motrin®) with Naproxen (Naprosyn®) because the results will be more side effects and not more pain relief.

You *can* take acetaminophen (Tylenol®) and one of the other NSAID medicines like Ibuprofen because they are not in the same family and they hit the pain differently. You can even add an opiate pain medicine to help ease the pain.

The main difference between COX-2 blockers and other NSAIDs is that these new drugs are less likely to develop intestinal side effects and are less likely to produce ulcers. COX-2 blockers also do not stop platelets from working to patch holes with clotting.

The protection COX-2 provides from stomach bleeding is removed when one takes aspirin as a preventative medicine. Many doctors advise their patients to take baby aspirin, or adult low dose aspirin (81 mg) daily not for pain relief, but to help prevent heart attack, stroke, colon cancer, and memory loss. If you take aspirin along with a COX-2 blocker, you must add a stomach protection medication like misoprostal (100–200 mcg twice a day), or omeprazole (20 mg once daily).

Aspirin

Aspirin is one of the oldest non-opiate pain medicines taken by mouth. The usual pain-fighting dose in an adult is 500 mg to 1000 mg by mouth every four to six hours, up to a total of 4000 mg a day. Aspirin should not be given to children under 12 who have cold or flu symptoms because it may cause a severe problem called Reye's syndrome. The children's dose for non-virus/flu/cold pain symptoms is 10–15 mg per kilogram of the child's weight.

In adults, low dose daily aspirin at 81 mg a day (one baby aspirin) has been shown to decrease strokes, heart attacks, and colon cancer. (This dose will not help pain in an adult.) Aspirin stops platelets (the small blood cells that plug up holes in blood vessels) from working and slows down blood clotting. This effect can last for up to two weeks. Your doctor may want you to stop aspirin two weeks before undergoing surgery or dental work. In any procedure that may cause bleeding, you want your blood clotting system to work at full capacity.

Aspirin can cause bleeding stomach ulcers and should not be taken if you have had a problem with ulcers in the past.

People who are allergic to aspirin, or who have nasal polyps, can get asthma, hives, and swelling from aspirin. You should avoid all medications with aspirin once you know that you are allergic.

Aspirin is available without a prescription and is inexpensive.

Other medications in the aspirin family that have fewer unwanted side effects and that can work longer than aspirin are:

- Trisalicylate (Trilisate®) 1000–1500 mg every eight to twelve hours

- Diflunisal (Dolobid®) 500 mg every eight to twelve hours
- Salsalate (Disalcid®) 500–750 mg one tablet every six hours or two tablets every twelve hours
- Sodium Salicylate (Uracel S®)
- Sodium thiosalicylate (Thiocyl®, Tusalv®)

Ibuprofen

Ibuprofen (Motrin®, Rufen, Nuprin®, Advil®, Medipren®, and many others) is available without prescription at the dose of 200 mg or lower. The adult dose is 200 mg–800 mg by mouth every six to eight hours for a maximum of 2,400 mg a day. The dose for children is 10 mg per kg body weight by mouth every six to eight hours.

Naproxen

Naproxen (Naprosyn®) and Naproxen Sodium (Anaprox®, Aleve®) is available without prescription at the dose of 220 mg (Aleve®). Prescription doses of over-the-counter Aleve® range from 230 mg to 500 mg every 12 hours up to a maximum of 1,250 mg a day.

Ketoprofen

Ketoprofen (Orudis®, Actron®, Orudis–K+®) is available without a prescription at the dose of 25 mg or lower. The adult dose is 25–75 mg every six–eight hours, for a maximum of 300 mg daily.

COX-2 Blockers

The main difference between these drugs called COX-2 blockers, or inhibitors, and the other NSAIDs is that they only block the chemical reaction that leads to inflammation in the body (COX-2), and do not block the chemical production of the protective stomach lining and platelets (COX-1). Since the major side effect of NSAIDs is bleeding stomach ulcer, these new drugs do not tend to produce ulcers. They also do not stop platelets from working to patch holes with clotting. There were increased numbers of heart attacks in patients taking refocoxib. Please ask your doctor if you are taking one of these medications.

COX2 Medications

- Partially *COX2* selective *NSAID*
  - etodolac (Lodine®) 200–400 mg twice to three times a day
  - eeodolac XL (Lodine XL®) 400–1200 mg daily
  - nabumetone (Relafen®) 1000 mg by mouth twice a day
- COX2 selective NSAID
  - celecoxib (Celebrax®) 100–200 mg. twice a day.

Ketoralac (Toradol®)

Ketoralac is the only NSAID that can be given directly in the vein or as a shot. It offers six hours of NSAID pain-fighting action. It has the same side effect profile as the other NSAIDs. The usual adult dose is 30 mg every six hours. Ketoralac is helpful for acute pain in emergency rooms. It can only be used for five continuous days at a time.

Other prescription NSAID names at the level of Ketoralac include:

diclofenac (Voltaren®, Arthrotec®, Cataflan®)
etodolac (Lodine®)
fenoprofen (Nalfon®)
flurbiprofen (Ansaid®)
meloxicam (Mobic®)
diflunisal (Dolobid®)
indomethacin (Indocin®)
isoxicam (Maxicam®)

ketoprofen (Orudis®, Oruvail®)
oxaprozin (Daypro®)
piroxicam (Feldene®)
meclofenamate (Meclomen®)
nabumetone (Relafen®)
sulindac (Clinoril®)
tolmetin (Tolectin®)

AGONIST-ANTAGONIST

Nalbuthine

Nalbuthine (Nubain®) is an injectable pain medication that blocks pain in the brain. It has several benefits:

- It does not slow down breathing.
- It does not cause itching.
- Its pain-fighting ability is near that of morphine in a ratio of 2 mg of nalbuthine equals 1 mg of morphine.

It does cause drowsiness and occasional nausea.

Nalbuthine will not fight pain after you reach the maximum dose of 20 mg every three hours. If pain is not controlled with the maximum dose, one must stop the nalbuthine and start treatment with morphine.

ANTI-SEIZURE MEDICATIONS

Anti-convulsants may be effective if pain is stabbing, burning, and intermittent, or does not respond to antidepressants. Again, start low, go slow.

The anti-seizure medication we have the most experience with is carbamazepine (Tegretol®), which is started at 100 mg daily and titrated slowly to 400–800 mg daily. Blood levels should be moni-

Dose by Weight for Common Non-opiates

Name	Dosage by Body weight		Notes
Acetaminophen (Tylenol®)	20 lbs	100 mg	Give every four hours; will block fever; will not upset stomach; does not block inflammation; maximum Adult dose 4000 mg every 24 hrs; Toxic doses damage the liver.
	30 lbs	150 mg	
	40 lbs	200 mg	
	50 lbs	250 mg	
	60 lbs	300 mg	
	70 lbs	350 mg	
	80 lbs	400 mg	
	90 lbs	450 mg	
	100 lbs	500 mg	
	120+	650 mg	
Ibuprofen (Advil®, Motrin®)	20 lbs	100 mg	Give every six to eight hours; will block a fever; may cause stomach ulcers; may damage kidneys; may increase bleeding; does block inflammation; maximum adult dose 3200 mg daily.
	30 lbs	150 mg	
	40 lbs	200 mg	
	50 lbs	250 mg	
	60 lbs	300 mg	
	70 lbs	350 mg	
	80 lbs	400 mg	
	90 lbs	450 mg	
	100 lbs	500 mg	
	120 lbs+	600 mg	
Aspirin	Adults only; 650 mg every 4–6 hours; 81 mg daily to slow clotting down.		All of the same notes as Ibuprofen; may cause Reye's syndrome in children, so do not use in children 12 and under.

tored, and there are risks of irritation to the bone marrow (which can show up as a slow-down in the normal production of red or white blood cells).

Other anticonvulsants such as phenytoin (Dilantin®), valproic acid (Depakote®), or clonazepam (Klonopin®) may also afford relief of pain. The newest of the anticonvulsants shown to be effective is gabapentin (Neurontin®). It is an attractive drug because its side effects seem to be less severe than those of the older anticonvulsants. It has been recently approved for treatment of pain that follows an outbreak of shingles—a type of pain that has been difficult to treat in the past.

ANTIDEPRESSANTS

Antidepressants are usually considered first-line treatment for neuropathic pain, and should be considered in cases of chronic pain from any cause. We have the most clinical experience with amitriptyline, but other tricyclic antidepressants (e.g., nortriptyline, imipramine, or doxepin), and heterocyclic (e.g., trazodone) may be effective also.

Studies of patients with diabetic neuropathy suggest that 60 percent of patients get 50 percent or more relief of pain from antidepressants. Analgesic effects occur sooner and at lower doses than the antidepressant effects. Treatment should begin with a low dose, e.g., 10–25 mg amitriptyline. Adjust the dose by 25 mg increments every three days to a maximum of 150 mg/day, or lower if the patient can't tolerate the side effects.

The dry mouth, difficulty urinating, blurred vision, and sedative effects of the older antidepressants may be significant, especially in severely debilitated patients and the elderly. Unfortunately, there is no evidence for the effectiveness of the newer antidepressants, such as fluoxetine (Prozac®) or sertraline (Zoloft®), which have fewer side effects. One recent study suggests that venlafaxine (Effexor®) may be effective in treating pain, independent of its antidepressant qualities.

Amitriptyline, nortriptyline, and desipramine have been established as analgesics, in addition to their antidepressant effects.

TRAMADOL

Tramadol (Ultram®) is a prescription-only pain medicine intended for people who have moderate to moderately severe chronic pain. Tramadol helps your body's system relieve pain in two important ways. First, Tramadol acts directly on parts of the brain and spinal cord to reduce the amount of pain. Second, it reduces the size of the pain signal passed from one nerve to another.

Tramadol works differently from a NSAID such as ibuprofen. It is also different from other pain medications, such as codeine or morphine.

Pain Matters

In this chapter you've learned what non-opiate medications are available for the treatment of pain. Many of these medications are available without prescription. They are the first line of defense against pain. Remember that all these medications can sometimes cause harmful side effects. Always check with your healthcare provider if you have any questions or concerns.

CHAPTER 9

Opiate Pain Medications

INTERNAL OPIATES

The body's own pain-blocking substances closely resemble opiate pain medications like morphine. The body makes brain chemicals (endorphins, among others) that block the pain signals in the brain and spinal cord. This built-in pain fighting system helps us tolerate painful injuries while they heal. The pain may be intense at first, but then the natural pain blockers begin to work.

Opiates also occur in nature in the opium poppy plant. The resin from the poppy flower is purified to give us the opiate class of pain-fighting medications that includes codeine, hydrocodone, hydromorphone, oxycodone, oxymorphone, meperidine, morphine, methadone, fentanyl, and propoxyphene. When the body is unable to keep up with the pain, these medical opiates can do the job.

COMMON ISSUES

Opiates have common side effects and carry the same precautions. They can cause you to become drowsy, unable to concentrate, and lightheaded. If you are on opiates, you should check with your doctor about driving, operating dangerous machinery, or taking other medications or substances (like allergy medications or alcohol) that cause drowsiness.

When you first go on opiates, nausea, dry mouth, and vomiting may occur. These symptoms often quiet down after a few doses, and they may improve just by your lying down. If the nausea continues, there are medications to help ease it.

Some opiates, especially morphine, cause the release of histamine in the skin, resulting in hives and itching. By taking the antihistamine diphenhydramine (Benadryl®), most patients can relieve this condition.

All opiates can slow the time it takes for food to be digested in the intestines, causing hard stools and constipation. This can be helped by taking a stool softener, drinking at least eight glasses of water daily, and eating a diet with a lot of fiber.

All opiates can cause physical dependence after several days of use. This is not addiction. This is a natural effect of the medication. When opiate medicines are stopped suddenly, the body will have a reaction called "withdrawal," causing stomach cramps, shaking, chills, rapid heart rate, diarrhea, sweats, goose bumps, runny nose, body aches, and dizziness. These withdrawal symptoms can be avoided by gradually decreasing your medication strength over several days. Your doctor should give you a taper schedule for decreasing the dose gradually.

All opiates can cause physical dependence after several days of use. This is not addiction.

Sometimes, patients and healthcare providers as well fear that opiates will cause addiction, which is defined as a compulsive use of a substance despite harm to the person. In fact, addiction happens in fewer than one out of 100 people being treated for pain.

Many people suffer pain needlessly because of their own fears and/or their doctor's fear of addiction.

Opiates can be given by intramuscular or subcutaneous injection. They reach a peak concentration in 30 minutes. A repeat dose can be given for unrelieved pain in 30 minutes. Opiates given by mouth reach a peak concentration in 60 to 90 minutes. Usually, your provider will order repeat doses of oral opiates on an "as needed" basis, every four to six hours. The long-acting oral opiates may take several hours to get the peak effect, but they last eight to twelve hours. The long-acting opiate should be given on schedule every 12 hours with a short acting opiate for breakthrough pain.

In fact, addiction happens in fewer than one out of 100 people being treated for pain.

For patients in severe pain, opiates should be given in the vein (intravenously) so that a peak effect is reached in six to 10 minutes. If the dose does not reduce the pain to a satisfactory level, a repeat increased dose can be given in 10 minutes.

Warning Signs of Drug Abuse and Addiction
Drug abuse is using pain medication to get high instead of fighting pain. The warning signs of drug abuse and addiction are:

- Constant use despite harm.
- Forging prescriptions.
- Avoiding treatment.
- Constant craving for the drug.
- Behavior that revolves around obtaining the drug.

Codeine

For oral dosage form (oral solution or tablets):

Adults: 15 to 60 mg (usually 30 mg) every three to six hours as needed.

Children: 0.5 mg per kilogram (kg) (0.2 mg per pound) of body weight every four to six hours as needed. Young children will probably take the oral solution, rather than tablets. Small doses may need to be measured by a special dropper instead of a teaspoon.

For injection dosage form:

Adults: 15 to 60 mg (usually 30 mg), injected into a muscle, a vein, or under the skin every four to six hours as needed.

Children: 0.5 mg per kg (0.2 mg per pound) of body weight, injected into a muscle or under the skin every four to six hours as needed.

Hydrocodone

For oral dosage form (syrup or tablets):

Adults: 5 to 10 milligrams (mg) every four to six hours as needed.

Children: 0.15 mg per kilogram (kg) (0.06 mg per pound) of body weight every six hours as needed.

Hydromorphone (Dilaudid®, Palladone®)

The clinical trials of sustained-release hydromorphone indicate that it has analgesic effects similar to those of morphine but with fewer side effects. This medication is safer than morphine for people with kidney disease because it does not build up in the blood if the kidneys aren't working well.

For oral dosage form (oral solution or tablets):
Adults: 2 or 2.5 milligrams (mg) every three to six hours as needed.
Children: Dose must be determined by your doctor.

For injection dosage form:
Adults: 1 or 2 mg, injected into a muscle or under the skin every three to six hours as needed. Some people may receive 0.5 mg, injected slowly into a vein every three hours as needed.
Children: Dose must be determined by your doctor.

For rectal suppository dosage form:
Adults: 3 mg every four to eight hours as needed.
Children: Dose must be determined by your doctor.

For long acting oral (extended-release tablets):
Adults only: Your doctor should determine your dosage, usually given once a day.

Oxycodone (Oxycontin®, Oxydose®, Oxyfast®, OxyIR®, Roxicodane®)

Oxycodone is more potent than morphine and has fewer side effects. A long-lasting version, introduced about five years ago, has quickly become the most popular opiate for treatment of chronic, non-cancer pain in the United States.

There have been occasional reports of agitation, sleeplessness, and dysphoria in patients taking high doses of oxycodone.

For oral dosage form (oral solution or tablets):
Adults: 5–15 milligrams (mg) every four to six hours as needed.
Children: Dose must be determined by your doctor. Children up to six years old will probably take the oral solution rather than tablets. Small doses may need to be measured by a special dropper instead of a teaspoon.

For long-acting oral dosage form (extended-release tablets):

Adults: Your doctor will determine the dose according to your individual needs. To be helpful, these medicines need to be taken two times a day at regularly scheduled times.

Children: Use and dose must be determined by your doctor.

For rectal suppository dosage form:

Adults: 10 to 40 mg three or four times daily.

Children: Dose must be determined by your doctor.

Oxymorphone (Numorphan®)

By injection:

Adults: 1 to 1.5 mg, injected into a muscle or under the skin every three to six hours as needed. Some patients may receive 0.5 mg, injected into a vein.

Children: Dose must be determined by your doctor.

Rectal suppository dosage form:

Adults: 5 mg every four to six hours as needed.

Children: Dose must be determined by your doctor.

Meperidine (Demerol®)

Oral dosage (syrup or tablets):

Adults: 50 to 150 mg (usually 100 mg) every three or four hours as needed.

Children: 1.1 to 1.76 mg per kg (0.44 to 0.8 mg per pound) of body weight, up to a maximum of 100 mg, every three or four hours as needed. Young children will probably take the syrup, rather than tablets. Small doses may need to be measured by a special dropper instead of a teaspoon.

By injection:

Adults: 50 to 150 mg (usually 100 mg), injected into a muscle or under the skin every three or four hours as needed. The medicine may also be injected continuously into a vein at a rate of 15 to 35 mg an hour.

Children: 1.1 to 1.76 mg per kg (0.44 to 0.8 mg per pound) of body weight, up to a maximum of 100 mg, injected into a muscle or under the skin every three or four hours as needed.

Meperidine, by injection in the muscle or in the vein, is effective for a few days of pain relief. The oral dosing is not helpful and there are much better opiates to take by mouth. Over time, meperidine can build up a brain toxin called nor-meperidine. This toxin can cause personality changes and even seizures. *It should not be used to treat chronic pain.* Ask your doctor about other medicines to use if you have chronic pain.

Morphine (Kadian®; MS Contin®, MSIR®, Oramorph SR®RMS; Roxanol®, Roxanol 100®)

Morphine is used to relieve moderate to severe pain. Morphine comes as a tablet, a capsule, a liquid, a controlled- or extended-release (long-acting) tablet, and as a sustained-release (long-acting) capsule, all taken by mouth. It also comes as a suppository to insert rectally.

The regular tablet, regular capsule, liquid, or suppository is usually taken every four hours as needed. The controlled- or extended-release tablet is taken every eight to twelve hours as needed. The sustained-release capsule is taken once or twice a day.

Morphine can cause the body to release histamine, which causes itching. This can be blocked with anti-histamine medications like diphenhydramine (Benadryl®). Morphine frequently causes nausea, but this can be blocked with anti-nausea medications like promethazine (Phenergan®).

Swallow the long-acting tablets and capsules whole. You may open the sustained-release capsules and sprinkle the entire contents on a small amount of applesauce immediately before eating. Do not chew, crush, or dissolve the pellets inside the capsules.

Shake the liquid well before measuring a dose. Ask your pharmacist for a specially marked measuring spoon that will help you measure exactly.

To insert a morphine suppository rectally, follow these steps:

1. Remove the wrapper.
2. Lie down on your left side and raise your right knee to your chest. (A left-handed person should lie on the right side and raise the left knee.)
3. Using your finger, insert the suppository into the rectum, about 1/2 to 1 inch for infants and children and 1 inch for an adult.
4. Stand up after about fifteen minutes. Wash your hands thoroughly and resume normal activities.

For short-acting oral dosage forms used for chronic pain:
Adults: At first, 10 to 30 mg every four hours. Your doctor will then adjust the dose according to your individual needs. If you have already been taking other narcotics to relieve severe chronic pain, your starting dose will depend on the amount of other narcotics you were taking daily.
Children: Dose must be determined by your doctor.

For long-acting oral dosage forms (extended-release capsules or tablets) used for severe, chronic pain (severe pain that lasts a long time):
Adults: Long-acting forms of morphine are usually used for patients who have already been receiving narcotics to relieve pain. The starting dose will depend on how much shorter-last-

ing a narcotic you have been receiving every day. Your doctor will adjust the dose according to that history and to your individual needs.

For these medicines to be helpful, they need to be taken twice a day at regularly scheduled times. Some people may need to take a short-acting form of morphine if pain occurs between doses of the long-acting medicine.

Children: Dose must be determined by your doctor.

By injection:

Adults: 5 to 20 mg (usually 10 mg), injected into a muscle or under the skin every four hours as needed. Some people may receive 4 to 10 mg, injected slowly into a vein. Morphine may also be injected continuously into a vein or under the skin at a rate that depends on the needs of the patient. This medicine may also be injected into the spinal area. The dose will depend on where and how the medicine is injected into the spinal area and on the needs of the patient.

Children: 0.1 to 0.2 mg per kg (0.04 or 0.09 mg per pound) of body weight, up to a maximum of 15 mg, injected under the skin every four hours as needed. Some patients may receive 0.05 to 0.1 mg per kg (0.02 to 0.04 mg per pound) of body weight, injected slowly into a vein.

By rectal suppository:

Adults: 10 to 30 mg every four to six hours as needed.

Children: Dose must be determined by your doctor.

Levorphanol and Methadone

By virtue of their long half-lives, methadone and levorphanol are also useful for treatment of chronic pain. Both have significant non-opiate effects that may contribute to their utility as pain relievers, especially for neuropathic pain. However, these drugs are generally reserved for second-line treatment because they are difficult to titrate and have delayed-onset side effects. To be effective, methadone must be administered at intervals six to eight hours shorter than its metabolic half-life (which is 15 to 90 hours). As serum levels of the drug increase, so does the risk of toxicity, primarily sedation.

Many U.S. physicians are under the impression that it is illegal to prescribe methadone without a license from the federal government, but that is the case only if methadone is used in a maintenance program for treatment of drug addiction. When prescribed for pain, methadone is subject to the same regulations as other high-potency opiates. One practical advantage of methadone and levorphanol is that they are both relatively inexpensive.

For levorphanol in oral dosage (tablets):
Adults: 2 mg. Some people with severe pain may need 3 or 4 mg.
Children: Dose must be determined by your doctor.

By injection
Adults: 2 mg, injected under the skin or into a vein. Some people may need 3 mg.
Children: Dose must be determined by your doctor.

For methadone in oral dosage:
Methadone (Dolophine®, Methadone®) is used to relieve severe pain. It is also used in treatment programs for people addicted to narcotics. Methadone comes as a tablet, dispersible tablet, liquid, and liquid concentrate to take by mouth. It is usually taken every three to four hours as needed for severe pain, or every six to eight hours for chronic pain. If you take methadone as part of a treatment program, your doctor will prescribe the dosing schedule that is best for you.

Dispersible tablets should be put in 3–4 ounces of liquid (e.g., water or citrus fruit juice) before use. The tablet should be completely dissolved in one minute.

When the methadone oral concentrate solution is used, the dose should first be mixed in 3–4 ounces of liquid (e.g., water or citrus fruit juice).

Oral solution:
Adults: 5 to 20 mg every four to eight hours.
Children: Dose must be determined by your doctor.

Oral tablet dosage form:
Adults: 2.5 to 10 mg every three or four hours as needed.
Children: Dose must be determined by your doctor.

By injection:
Adults: 2.5 to 10 mg, injected into a muscle or under the skin, every three or four hours as needed.
Children: Dose must be determined by your doctor.

Fentanyl (Duragesic®, Sublimaze®)

Fentanyl, a derivative of meperidine, was specifically designed to substitute for morphine in operations when anesthesia is used. It is fast-acting. More importantly, it is hundreds of times more powerful than morphine. Microgram amounts, administered by a skin patch, can provide pain relief for up to 72 hours. Follow the directions on applying the patch and remove them at the proper time.

Oral trans mucosal fentanyl citrate is an effective and well-tolerated treatment for the long-term management of patients with severe pain. This medication is in a lollipop form, to dissolve slowly through the lining of the mouth.

Propoxyphene (Darvon®)

Oral dosage (capsules, oral suspension, or tablets):

Adults: Propoxyphene comes in two different forms, propoxyphene hydrochloride (Darvon®) and propoxyphene napsylate. One hundred mg of propoxyphene napsylate provides the same amount of pain relief as 65 mg of propoxyphene hydrochloride. The dose of propoxyphene hydrochloride is 65 mg every four hours as needed, up to a maximum of 390 mg a day. The dose of propoxyphene napsylate is 100 mg every four hours as needed, up to a maximum of 600 mg a day.

Propoxyphene can produce buildup of a toxic byproduct that can cause seizures.

Pain Matters

Opiates are effective painkillers that may also have unwelcome side effects. By taking preventive action and watching for symptoms, your doctor and you can maximize the benefits while minimizing the side effects.

Opiates should not be feared by patients or providers. They are simply an extension of the body's own built-in opiate pain-fighting system. Properly used, opiates offer powerful relief to people in severe pain.

CHAPTER 10

Non-medication Pain Treatments

Not all pain treatment depends on prescriptions. In this chapter, we will walk you through treatments that are often used alone or along with medication.

PHYSICAL THERAPY

Heat

Most of us have used a heating pad to soothe aching muscles. We use it because it works. The use of a heating pad, hot pack, or paraffin wax has been clinically proven to:

- Reduce joint stiffness.
- Reduce muscle spasm.
- Increase circulation to aid in healing.
- Temporarily reduce pain levels.

Superficial heat (heat that comes through contact with the skin) is an economical treatment choice that can be used in almost any setting and requires little instruction. Superficial heat is an effective addition to other pain reduction therapies, such as therapeutic exercise, therapeutic massage, and chiropractic adjustment.

Heating pads typically use electric current to heat coils within the pad. *Hot packs* are most commonly used at home and contain a synthetic material that is heated in the microwave. *Paraffin treatments* consist of wax heated to its melting point, applied in layers, and allowed to solidify. Each method delivers heat through contact with the skin. Treatment times range from 15 to 30 minutes. Heating pads and hot packs are effective in the treatment of specific or large body areas. Paraffin is most often used for treating the hands.

In order to reduce the risk of burns or injury, we need to be careful how we use superficial heat. A person should never go to sleep using a heating pad, because blistering or burns can occur. Also, the area being treated should be monitored both during and after treatment to insure that the heat source hasn't caused blistering or skin irritation.

If you are a hemophiliac (prone to increased bleeding) or are taking steroid or blood-thinning medications, you should consult with your healthcare provider before starting superficial heat treatment. Likewise, people whose sense of feeling is impaired or gone, as well as people with diminished mental capabilities, should use extreme caution with heat. Burns can occur before you realize that you are being burned.

Warning: *Acute injuries that need healing should not be treated with heat. Heat causes an increase in blood flow to the injured area, and the increase will cause further swelling and delayed healing.*

Therapeutic Ultrasound

Therapeutic ultrasound is a form of deep heat that penetrates one to one-and-a-half inches below the skin. It delivers many of the same benefits as superficial heat (increasing circulation, decreasing joint stiffness and muscle spasms), and also delivers a more permanent reduction in pain levels.

Ultrasound works like this: Electrical current, passed through a crystal within the treatment applicator, causes high frequency sound waves to be generated. These waves penetrate the skin via a topical medium (gel or water), and in this way heat specific internal joints and tissues without heating the skin. Therapeutic ultrasound is typically used along with other pain reduction treatments, such as superficial heat, therapeutic exercise, and chiropractic adjustment.

Therapeutic ultrasound is typically performed by a licensed physical therapist in a clinic or home setting. Most health insurance plans cover treatment if a healthcare provider orders that treatment for a specific injury or disease. Therapeutic ultrasound should never be performed over a cardiac pacemaker, the abdomen of a pregnant woman, or a cancerous tumor. People with impaired or absent sensation or impaired circulation should consult their health care provider before starting treatment. People with metal implants, such as joint replacements, screws, or plates, can be treated with therapeutic ultrasound at specific settings, but they should tell the treating attendant about these implements *before* starting treatment.

Cold or Cryotherapy

Cryotherapy is the therapeutic use of cold (either a cold pack or ice massage) after an acute injury or surgery. Such treatment inhibits nerve transmission, reduces circulation and inflammation, and minimizes pain. Cryotherapy can be used with therapeutic exercises to reduce exercise soreness, discomfort, and swelling.

Cold packs can be purchased at the local drug store. They contain a gel-like substance that allows for repeated refreezing. Homemade cold packs using frozen peas, ice cubes or crushed ice are just as good, but they tend to leak.

Cold packs are the preferred choice for the treatment of large body areas. They are used for 15 to 20 minutes or until numbness is achieved. Ice massage consists of the direct application of ice (usually frozen in a paper cup with the sides peeled back) to the affected area for three to four minutes, or until the area is numb. Ice massage is best used in the treatment of a specific, localized area.

Cryotherapy is an economical treatment choice that can be used in almost any setting with minimal instruction or training.

People with blocked circulation, and people who are hypersensitive to cold (Raynaud's phenomenon) are not candidates for cryotherapy. People with impaired or absent circulation should consult with their healthcare provider prior to initiating cryotherapy.

Massage

Muscle massage can increase blood flow and reduce muscle spasms, thus helping a person relax. Massage helps distract the mind from the pain. A friend or family member can massage your neck and back muscles to help ease headache, neck pain, or back pain. A physical therapist can help you learn muscle massage techniques that help relieve muscle spasm and aid relaxation. There are massaging mechanical chairs that can help ease back pain. (For more information, see the section on therapeutic massage in Chapter 13.)

Biofeedback

Electrical biofeedback became popular in the 1970's with the growing interest in mind/body connection. Early studies focused on a person's ability to cause a physical change in his or her body in response to an external monitoring device. Electrode sensors placed on a muscle would indicate muscle tension via electrical impulses. Those impulses would then generate a visual signal or audible tone. As a person learned to consciously relax the muscle, the signal or tone would lessen. In this way a person learned to monitor muscle tension and apply relaxation techniques against it.

Today, biofeedback is widely used in the treatment of weakened or injured muscles. Through visual or tonal cues from the biofeedback unit, a person can consciously focus on tightening/strengthening that specific muscle group during exercise.

Thermal biofeedback uses sensors that monitor body temperature changes. This type of biofeedback is most commonly used with circulatory ailments, such as migraine headaches, high blood pressure, and Raynaud's phenomenon. Like electrical biofeedback, thermal biofeedback allows you to self-monitor and regulate your circulatory system.

Biofeedback must be taught by a trained professional, and successful training requires both time and motivation. Once you've completed your training, portable units are available for home use.

Traditional health insurance plans typically cover treatment if ordered by a healthcare provider for a specific injury or disease process. Effectiveness of this therapy for pain relief depends on your willingness to practice the biofeedback techniques consistently and regularly. People who are chronically depressed or who are not motivated to improve are not appropriate candidates for biofeedback therapy.

Transcutaneous Electrical Nerve Stimulation

Transcutaneous electrical nerve stimulation (TENS) has been clinically proven to successfully manage acute injury and surgical pain, though it has been less successful in the long-term management of chronic pain. Electrical stimulation is delivered from a battery-operated unit through electrodes placed over the affected area. Most people feel this low-level stimulation as a tingling sensation. The TENS unit is portable and can be carried in a pocket or clipped to a belt.

TENS reduces the level of pain in two ways. The first way is referred to as the "Gate Theory," in which the stimulus provided by the unit blocks nerves that carry pain signals to the brain. The second way is through the release of endorphins from the brain in response to the stimulation of the nerves, generating a "natural high." With a referral from a healthcare provider for a specific injury or disease process, most traditional health insurance plans cover treatment

Use of TENS is typically taught by a licensed physical therapist in a clinic or home setting. Usually, one session is enough to teach you to use TENS at home, where you can use the unit as often or steadily as you need to.

TENS should not be used when you are taking a shower, and it's a good thing to check the skin under the electrodes to be sure there's no irritation. People with impaired or absent sensation are not good candidates for TENS use. Likewise, people with diminished mental capability who don't clearly understand the use of the unit usually don't benefit from TENS.

Therapeutic Exercise

Study after study has shown the health benefits of regular physical activity and exercise. Benefits of exercise include:

- Improved heart and lung functions.
- Increased strength and endurance.
- Improved immune system function.
- Reduced stress.
- Greater control of such chronic diseases as diabetes, obesity, osteoporosis, and arthritis.

Actually, therapeutic exercise speeds up your healing and your return to normal function, especially when it is used with other pain reduction treatments, such as superficial heat, therapeutic ultrasound, and therapeutic massage.

Unfortunately, with an injury, surgery, or flare-up of a chronic illness, most people stop exercising because they think that exercise will cause more pain. Actually, therapeutic exercise speeds up your healing and your return to normal function, especially when it is used with other pain reduction treatments, such as superficial heat, therapeutic ultrasound, and therapeutic massage.

Therapeutic exercise is initiated in three stages. The first stage is designed to help you improve flexibility and movement of the painful area. In this early phase of healing, gentle stretching and yoga-type movements are used. All movements are done slowly and within your pain tolerance. The slogan, "No pain, no gain," doesn't apply here. Forcing movement can actually cause further injury and delay healing.

The second stage of therapeutic exercise focuses on improving strength to restore function of the affected area. People do this by lifting weights, or by using a large rubber band called a "theraband" to add resistance to movement. In using weights or a theraband, start off easy, with light weights or low resistance, so as to avoid risk of re-injury or increased pain.

As your strength improves, the number of repetitions should be increased, and only when that new level is established, the weight or resistance may also be increased. As an example, let's look at the use of a leg weight to improve strength. You might start with two-pound weight, and do ten repetitions of the exercise.

Once you are able to do several sets of twenty repetitions using the two-pound weight, the weight is increased to three or four pounds, and the number of repetitions is decreased to allow you to adjust to the greater weight.

The final stage of therapeutic exercise focuses on conditioning and endurance. Aerobic activities, such as walking, jogging, swimming, and bicycling, are some of the conditioning exercises you can choose from. As with strengthening exercises, start slowly and don't try to exercise too long. Gradually, as you get back your strength and conditioning, you will progress to more strenuous activity. An example of this principle: Start with a walking program of 10 minutes daily, progressing to 30 minutes daily, until, as a final goal, you can jog 20 to 30 minutes every day.

Therapeutic exercise instruction is typically performed by a licensed physical therapist working in a clinic or home setting. Traditional health insurance plans typically cover treatment with a referral from a healthcare provider for a specific injury or disease.

If you are being treated with therapeutic exercise, you will be given a written home exercise program to help you to continue doing the exercises daily. The program will also prepare you for transition to independent exercise.

Success in therapeutic exercise depends on maintaining pain at the lowest level possible. Adequate pain medication and the use of other pain-reduction treatments are essential in order for a person with serious pain to be able to continue with any exercise program.

People who aren't motivated to perform the exercises consistently will not benefit from this treatment. People with diminished mental capability will need ongoing supervision to ensure that exercises are done correctly and consistently.

Before starting any therapeutic exercise program, it is always a good idea to consult your healthcare provider.

MIND/BODY THERAPY

Mind/body therapy is designed to help you take your mind off the pain. Thinking about how bad the pain is makes it worse. You become fearful, tense your muscles, and increase the pain. That's why it is helpful to get your mind off of the pain.

Here are some methods to try:

Imagery

Imagery has been used in spiritual and healing ceremonies since the time of Aristotle, and can be considered the basis for all mind/body interactions. Clinical studies have shown that the use of focused imagery techniques can bring about significant physical changes in blood chemistry, heart/breathing rates, and brain activity.

Athletes use imagery before a competition, reviewing the event from start to finish in order to "practice" their response in advance. Cancer patients being treated with chemotherapy often use imagery to reduce nausea or to picture their cancer cells being destroyed. Imagery is also used with relaxation therapy, allowing a person to be in a fully relaxed and focused state of mind as he or she practices using imagery.

Two specific types of imagery are used to treat pain. *Pain-transforming imagery* allows you to change your response to pain even when the actual physical cause does not change. *Pain incompatible imagery* allows you to transcend your pain, in essence taking you mentally to a place where there is no pain.

A trained professional is necessary to teach specific imagery techniques, but once you've learned them, you can perform the techniques on your own, in any quiet setting.

Imagery is not recommended for persons suffering from diabetes, because changes in blood chemistry can occur and adversely affect blood sugar. Likewise, persons with diminished mental capability may have difficulty following instructions and are generally not good candidates for imagery therapy. Before starting either treatment, people suffering from seizures or chronic depression should consult their healthcare provider about any potential unwelcome side effects of brainwave changes that can occur during imagery.

Relaxation Therapy

The principles of relaxation therapy were established almost 100 years ago by Edmund Jacobson, although use of relaxation techniques to reduce pain has been documented for thousand of years. In his studies, Jacobson found that a person could increase muscle tension with the mere thought of movement.

Jacobson theorized that over time this accumulation of muscle tension could lead to poor sleep and disease. So he developed a series of techniques designed to help the patient consciously monitor each area of the body, with the goal to decrease unwanted muscle tension periodically throughout the day.

Training to learn Jacobson's method was time-consuming, and much simpler variations in these techniques have been developed. Today, most researchers agree that relaxation therapy helps reduce muscle tension, and also helps in the management of high blood pressure. People using these techniques experience less stress and lower pain levels during relaxation therapy.

Today, relaxation techniques have been expanded to include both deep breathing and muscle tension reduction techniques. Quiet music can also help enhance relaxation. Typically, relaxation therapy is used with other therapies in the treatment of pain. Relaxation therapy techniques are easy to master, and, once learned, they can be performed independently in any quiet setting.

Relaxation therapy is usually taught by a trained professional, but basic techniques can be learned through book or a video. Persons with diminished mental capability may have difficulty mastering relaxation techniques. There are no other precautions or limitations.

Here is an exercise you might try. Start by getting comfortable, either sitting or lying down, and listening to soothing music in a quiet room. Get in a comfortable position. Make a fist and then release you fingers and concentrate on letting them go limp. Tense your arm muscles and then let them go limp. Tense your shoulders; then let them go limp. Tense your neck; then let it go limp. Scrunch your face muscles; then let them go limp. Tense your toes and feet; then let them go limp. Tense your leg muscles; then let them go limp. Tense your stomach and let it go limp.

All of your muscles should be relaxed. If any feel tense, repeat tightening them and letting them go until they are relaxed. Think of a calm place that you have visited like a beach or park. Meditate on your favorite scriptures, song, or event.

Biofeedback can help train you to relax.

Meditation

Meditation has been used in Eastern medicine and by some religions for thousand of years, but only in the last 25 to 30 years has meditation gained widespread acceptance in the Western medical community. Much like relaxation therapy, meditation has been shown to reduce heart rate, blood pressure, and breathing rates, and also to reduce levels of stress and pain.

While both meditation and relaxation therapy focus primarily on reducing muscle tension, meditation also has secondary benefits. It encourages you to concentrate your thoughts, and the mental clarity that results is what allows physical changes to occur. All forms of meditation follow more or less the same format: You practice in a quiet place with limited distractions, assume a comfortable/relaxed position, and identify a focal point (an object, sound or even your own breath).

Channeling all mental activity on that single focal point is believed to allow the mind to "reset itself" apart from the stress and anxiety of daily life. This, in turn, translates into measurable changes in muscle tone, blood chemistry, cardiovascular responses, and helps bring on a feeling of emotional well-being.

As with relaxation therapy, meditation is often used in conjunction with other therapies in the treatment of pain. Meditation requires an instructor in the beginning, but once you've learned the technique, you can practice by yourself in any quiet setting. For it to work, meditation practice must be consistent and regular, and requires that you can focus on a single object or mental activity.

Meditation is not recommended for persons suffering from diabetes, because it can bring about changes in blood chemistry that adversely affect blood sugar. Likewise, before starting treatment, persons suffering from seizures or chronic depression should consult their healthcare provider about any potential side effects of brain wave changes that occur during meditation.

Prayer

Many people with pain find comfort in prayer and meditation on favorite scripture verses. Here are some Bible scriptures that may be of comfort:

He was despised and rejected by men, a man of pain, and familiar with sickness. Like one from whom men hide their faces he was despised, and we esteemed him not. Surely he took up our sickness and carried our pain, yet we considered him stricken by God, smitten by him and afflicted. **Isaiah 53:3.** *(Amplified Bible).*

Jabez was more honorable than his brothers. His mother had named him Jabez, saying, "I gave birth to him in pain" [10]. Jabez cried out to the God of Israel, "Oh, that you would bless me and *enlarge my territory! Let your hand be with me, and keep me from harm so that I will be free from pain." And God granted his request. **1 Chron. 4:9–10** (New International Version)*

*Jesus went throughout Galilee, teaching in their synagogues, preaching the good news of the kingdom, and healing every disease and sickness among the people [24]. News about him spread all over Syria, and people brought to him all who were ill with various diseases, those suffering severe pain, the demon-possessed, those having seizures, and the paralyzed, and he healed them. **Matthew 4:23–24** (New International Version)*

*A woman giving birth to a child has pain because her time has come; but when her baby is born she forgets the anguish because of her joy that a child is born into the world. **John 16:21** (New International Version)*

Praise the Lord, O my soul; all my inmost being, praise his holy name.
Praise the Lord, O my soul, and forget not all his benefits—
who forgives all your sins and heals all your diseases,
who redeems your life from the pit and crowns you with love and compassion,
who satisfies your desires with good things so that your youth is renewed like the eagle's.
The Lord works righteousness and justice for all the oppressed.
He made known his ways to Moses, his deeds to the people of Israel:
The Lord is compassionate and gracious, slow to anger, abounding in love.
He will not always accuse, nor will he harbor his anger forever;
he does not treat us as our sins deserve or repay us according to our iniquities.
For as high as the heavens are above the earth so great is his love

for those who fear him; as far as the east is from the west, so far has he removed our transgressions from us. **Psalm 103** *(New International Version)*

Trust in the Lord with all your heart and lean not on your own understanding; in all your ways acknowledge him, and he will make your paths straight. Do not be wise in your own eyes; fear the Lord and shun evil. This will bring health to your body and nourishment to your bones. **Proverbs 3:5** *(New International Version)*

When you lie down, you will not be afraid; when you lie down your sleep will be sweet. **Proverbs 3:24** *(New International Version)*

My son, pay attention to what I say; listen closely to my words. Do not let them out of your sight, keep them within your heart; for they are life to those who find them, and health (medicine) to a man's whole body. **Proverbs 4:20** *(New International Version)*

Reckless words pierce like a sword, but the tongue of the wise brings healing. **Proverbs 12:18** *(New International Version)*

Pleasant words are as a honeycomb, sweet to the soul, and health to the bones. **Proverbs 16:24** *(New International Version)*

A cheerful heart is good medicine, but a crushed spirit dries up the bones. **Proverbs 17:22** *(New International Version)*

When he came down from the mountainside, large crowds followed him. A man with leprosy came and knelt before him and said, "Lord, if you are willing, you can make me clean."

Jesus reached out his hand and touched the man. "I am willing," he said. "Be clean!" Immediately he was cured of his leprosy. Then Jesus said to him, "See that you don't tell anyone. But go, show yourself to the priest and offer the gift Moses commanded, as a testimony to them. . . ."

When Jesus came into Peter's house, he saw Peter's mother-in-law lying in bed with a fever. He touched her hand and the fever left her, and she got up and began to wait on him.

When evening came, many who were demon-possessed were brought to him, and he drove out the spirits with a word and healed all the sick. This was to fulfill what was spoken through the prophet Isaiah: "He took up our infirmities and carried our diseases." **Matthew 8:1–17** *(New International Version)*

One day Peter and John were going up to the temple at the time of prayer—at three in the afternoon. Now a man crippled from birth was being carried to the temple gate called Beautiful, where he was put every day to beg from those going into the temple courts. When he saw Peter and John about to enter, he asked them for money. Peter looked straight at him, as did John. Then Peter said, "Look at us!" So the man gave them his attention, expecting to get something from them. Then Peter said, "Silver or gold I do not have, but what I have I give you. In the name of Jesus Christ of Nazareth, walk." Taking him by the right hand, he helped him up, and instantly the man's feet and ankles became strong. He jumped to his feet and began to walk. Then he went with them into the temple courts, walking and jumping, and praising God. When all the people saw him walking and praising God they recognized him as the same man who used to sit begging at the temple gate called Beautiful, and they were filled with wonder and amazement at what had happened to him. **Acts 3:2** *(New International Version)*

Hypnosis

Over the centuries, hypnosis has been used by many cultures as part of religious and healing ceremonies. During the 1930s and

40s, Dr. Milton Erickson, who theorized that our mental processes had a direct effect on both our physical and emotional well-being, conducted clinical studies involving the use of hypnosis as a way of verifying his thesis.

Dr. Erickson used a hypnotic procedure referred to as "discovery and suggestion," and he found that, with its help, he could help a person resolve specific stresses or conflicts.

Hypnosis requires you to clear your mind, relax mental control, and reduce awareness of external noise/stimulus, while focusing on a particular goal. While the subject is in this relaxed state, the therapist gives suggestions to support the subject's goal—say, to stop smoking, or to lose weight.

A person undergoing hypnotic technique remains awake throughout the treatment session and will not agree to suggestions that are contrary to their core beliefs or desires.

Hypnosis has been clinically demonstrated to reduce all levels of pain to some degree. Hypnosis works by changing your psychological response to pain, and, by doing so, it helps to relieve the anxiety, stress, and suffering that goes with chronic pain. "The pain," a patient might say, "is still there, but hypnosis has given me better mental ways of dealing with it."

Hypnosis has been clinically demonstrated to reduce all levels of pain to some degree.

As with meditation, for hypnosis to work, you must be able to channel mental energy toward your goal—in this case, the goal of easing pain. You must also be willing to practice consistently, and on a regular schedule.

To learn self-hypnosis, you first must be trained by a professional. After that, you are able to practice the same techniques at home.

Before trying hypnotic techniques, persons suffering from seizures or chronic depression should consult their healthcare provider about any potential bad side effects of brain-wave changes that occur during hypnosis. Persons with diminished mental capability may have reduced success with hypnotic techniques.

YOGA

Yoga originated in India over 3,000 years ago as part of a natural medicine system referred to as the "Ayurvedic" system. Yoga is a series of techniques designed to connect the mind and body. In fact, the Sanskrit word for yoga is translated as "union." Just as a balanced *qi (chi)*, or life force, is an essential element of Chinese medicine, yoga aims for a balance of the physical, mental, and spiritual components of a person's being. A recent study reported that over two million Americans routinely perform some type of yoga activity as part of their exercise routine.

The most popular form of yoga practiced in the United States is called Hatha yoga, which is comprised of three separate practices:

Asanas: Eighty-five different postures and exercises designed to realign the skeletal system, improve blood flow, and promote relaxation.

Pranayama: Breathing techniques designed to restore the balance between the mind and body-life forces.

Dhyana: Meditation practices designed to promote relaxation and clarify the mind.

Yoga postures, exercises, and breathing techniques can be used after an injury or surgery to reduce pain and improve flexibility and movement.

All techniques are performed in a slow, deliberate manner and can be done by people of all ages. Yoga techniques are usually taught by a trained practitioner, and classes for all levels are often held at health clubs and community centers.

Many books and videos available on the market can instruct you in yoga techniques at home. As with all exercise, before you start in a yoga program, if you've had a recent surgery or injury, talk to your healthcare provider about the pluses and minuses of yoga in your particular case.

Yoga practice for pain treatment requires your serious willingness to practice in a disciplined way. People who aren't strongly motivated aren't likely to get great benefits from yoga.

Distraction

Another way to get you mind off of the pain is to occupy your time with activities you enjoy. Here are a few types of activities to try.

Music

Listening to your favorite music can help your body relax, so you can take your mind off the pain. It also helps reduce blood pressure and stress, and to calm fear. Pick selections that relax and soothe. You can carry a portable CD or MP3 player on your belt, so that the music is there to draw on when you need it.

Many libraries have music collections from which you can borrow for free. Try them out, and decide which of them you might want to buy to listen to at home. Music is a strong tool; make it part of your "distraction toolbox."

Games

Video, card, and board games can distract your mind from pain and offer you an enjoyable break. Pick games that are fun for you and get you involved with others. If you like electronic games, there are plenty of inexpensive and portable ones on the market. Walk the toy isle at your local department store and pick up a few games to play. (A special advantage of board games is that they bring the family together for fun and interaction.) Join a bridge or chess group at your local community center or church.

Hobbies

If you already have a hobby, keep at it. What better way to take your mind away from the pain! If you don't already have a hobby, consider developing one. Hobbies can be a pleasurable distraction.

Naturally, if you are ready to start on a new hobby, pick one that doesn't make your pain worse. You have a wide range of choices. Many local community organizations, high schools, and colleges offer evening classes in photography, painting, ceramics, gardening, investing, writing, or travel. In hobbies you'll find a low-cost way to fill two needs: You'll distract yourself from your pain, and you're likely to make new friends.

Work

Getting back to work can improve your pain and speed your recovery. After all, work too can be a distraction, something you can lose yourself in, so that there's no place for the pain. If your pain is so severe that it keeps you from work, talk to your provider about physical exercises and retraining in pain management. Sometimes that works to make pain tolerable where it was intolerable before.

Many states offer vocational rehabilitation programs to retrain you if you've been forced to leave your job because of pain. You might also want to consider getting a degree or training in a field that offers more employment options and benefits.

Once you have that job, make sure you enjoy going to work. You will enjoy it, if your work is meaningful to you, by giving you the satisfaction of doing a good job on a daily basis.

Exercise

Walking and swimming are excellent distractions from pain, and such exercise will increase your body's pain-fighting substances (endorphins). Exercise has other benefits as well. It helps your muscle tone and stamina. It also helps keep your weight down, so it reduces bone and joint pain.

Finding ways to exercise shouldn't be a problem. Start off by walking to places nearby that you used to drive to. Before long you'll find that walking is something you crave. It's good both solo and with friends. In bad weather, try walking in your local shopping mall. Many malls allow walkers before and after store closing time.

Swimming is an excellent form of exercise that doesn't damage joints. Other sports that are relatively easy on the body include golf, bowling, bicycling, and rowing.

If you're looking for organized activity, join your community Y or local health club that has exercise facilities and equipment. Try to set a routine that becomes a habit for life.

Before starting an exercise program, talk to your provider for advice as to what program they think would work best for you.

Pain Matters

There are many non-medication methods you can use to reduce pain. Not all are effective in every situation or for every person, but, in conversation with your provider, you can find out which one is likely to work best for you. Many of these techniques cost you nothing and the benefits can be great. People who fight pain most effectively have more than one tool in their toolbox. It's simply a question of adding the tools that work for you.

CHAPTER 11

Pain Procedures

You and your healthcare providers have a variety of effective ways to help you control pain, as you've seen in the last three chapters. But when pain can't be controlled with the medications and treatments we have already described, more invasive treatments may be necessary. Such procedures, upon recommendation of your primary-care provider, are usually performed by specialists. The procedures are more costly and carry greater risk, but the outcome can be miraculous when the pain is reduced or even removed.

NERVE BLOCKS

When your pain is caused by a pinched nerve, or is localized, the nerves that carry the pain signals can be blocked by injecting long-acting numbing medications, like bupivacaine. This procedure is usually done by pain specialist doctors or anesthesiologists. An injection of bupivacaine can provide pain relief, at least for several days or even weeks. The injections may be repeated. Usually, these injections are done in the pain specialist's office. They don't require hospitalization.

INJECTIONS

When pain is caused by muscle or joint inflammation, like bursitis, an injection in the area may offer pain relief for several days or weeks. Family practice, orthopedic and rheumatology doctors do the injections in their offices. If your clinician isn't trained to do injections, ask for a referral to a specialist who can.

The medicine injected is usually a steroid to calm the inflammation, and a numbing medication to block the pain. Injection into joints over time can cause damage, so keep track of the number of injections, and talk with your doctor about the best schedule.

A risk you face with this procedure is the injection of germs into your joint. That could cause a serious infection that can destroy the joint space, so it requires treatment with antibiotics, usually administered in the vein (intravenous) in the hospital. There are good ways to minimize these risks: first, by making sure the needle is kept sterile, and, second, by keeping the skin area where the catheters were placed, sterile and protected. If the injection is done using a sterile technique, with careful cleansing of the skin and the use of sterile gloves, the risk of infection is minimized.

PAIN PUMPS

Pain medication, usually an opiate, can be pumped slowly into your bloodstream or spinal cord through a catheter. The pumps are small computers the size of a pocket radio, and they can be programmed to give a safe dose of medication on schedule around the clock. The pump is most often used during and after surgery for pain control. Pain medicine delivered in the spinal cord offers good pain control with minimal side effects. Pain pumps are also used when all other pain treatment methods have failed.

Like injection, pain pumps have their risks of infection if germs are injected into the spinal fluid or blood stream. Infections of this kind require hospitalization and antibiotics. Infection can be minimized by keeping the area of the skin where the catheter enters sterile and protected. Pain pumps are usually placed and managed by pain management specialists or anesthesiologists.

SURGERY

When pain is related to a slipped disc, a pinched nerve, cancer, or arthritis, surgery may offer the best treatment for pain relief. Surgeons can even cut the nerves that continually carry the wrong pain message.

Surgery is a last resort. For as long as possible your doctor should use medications to control the pain. Only in cases where your medication treatment fails will your doctor refer you to a surgeon.

Pain Matters

The procedures we've described in this chapter are usually reserved for people who suffer chronic pain and have found no relief in any of the first-line treatments. If you are in such a situation, work with your doctor to find a specialist with whom you can discuss these options. You want someone with a lot of experience, willing to listen to you, and ready to tell you both the benefits and risks of these therapies.

CHAPTER 12

Alternative Treatments, Herbal Medicines, and Nutritional Supplements

Alternative treatments are treatments not part of the traditional medical office or hospital, but these practices have been helpful for many people with pain. The medical profession calls these therapies "Complementary and Alternative Medicine" or CAM. The U.S. National Institutes of Health (NIH) has now established a National Center for CAM, where new treatments are tested for safety and effectiveness. See their website at *www.altmed.od.nih.gov*.

Be on guard against people who are trying to make money by selling you treatments that don't work. One watchdog resource is *www.quackwatch.com*. In this chapter, we discuss CAM treatments that have been shown to work.

CHIROPRACTIC INTERVENTION

While physical manipulation of joints has been a documented healing technique for thousands of years, chiropractic techniques as currently performed were established in the early 1900's. Today, chiropractors are the second largest group of primary healthcare providers in the United States. They provide almost 70 percent of all back care treatments, and enjoy one of the highest satisfaction ratings of all healthcare professionals.

Chiropractic care is based on the theory of misalignment of the body, specifically the bones around the spinal cord, causes pressure and inflammation to the nerves coming out of the spine. This nerve damage can cause pain, weakness, muscle spasm, numbness, headaches, and even loss of function. Through manual adjustments and manipulations to these bones, the chiropractor works to realign the spine, so that nerves can begin to heal.

Other therapies, such as superficial heat, therapeutic ultrasound, and therapeutic exercise, may be used along with chiropractic techniques to reduce pain and restore you to normal activity.

Clinical studies confirm the effectiveness of chiropractic intervention in the treatment of back and neck pain. Further wide-scale studies are being delayed, in part because of the long-standing hostility between the conventional medical and the chiropractic communities. Still, as the concept of holistic care becomes more prevalent in the management of pain, greater coordination of care between all healthcare providers is bound to develop, with the aim of more successful, cost-effective treatment.

Chiropractic care is provided in a clinic setting by a licensed Doctor of Chiropractics. Traditional health insurance plans often cover the cost of treatment. Persons suffering from bone disorders, such as fractures, osteoporosis, or infection from tumors, are not appropriate candidates for chiropractic manipulation. Likewise, persons suffering from an impaired circulatory system, severe systemic arthritis, or metabolic disorders should consult their healthcare provider before starting any treatment.

ACUPUNCTURE/ACUPRESSURE

Acupuncture has been a mainstay in Chinese medicine for thousands of years. This treatment system is based on the belief that a person's body is inherently balanced in terms of life force, or *qi* (pronounced *chee*). When this balance is disrupted, illness and disease may occur. Through the use of acupuncture or acupressure, this balance of life force is restored, and the person is returned to optimal health.

Practitioners of acupuncture have identified twelve energy pathways (meridians) that run through the body. Each meridian is connected to a specific internal organ, and each contains hundreds of acupuncture points that correspond to nerve endings. In the practice of acupuncture, these points, hypersensitive to pressure, are usually stimulated with a needle, though they can also be stimulated with heat or electrical current, or through manual pressure.

Stimulation of individual acupuncture points is believed to treat specific imbalances within the body, and treatment is modified as symptoms change or vanish. Clinical studies confirm that stimulation of the acupuncture points causes an increase in nerve activity within the corresponding pathway, and that the activity changes the blood chemistry.

Further studies are under way to understand fully how these bodily responses to acupuncture and acupressure translate into decreased pain levels and improved/restored function. What we do know is that they work. Acupressure techniques are often incorporated in therapeutic massage to yield greater pain relief.

Acupuncture is performed by a licensed and highly trained professional in a clinic setting. Acupuncture treatment is not appropriate for:

- Young children.
- Pregnant women.
- Persons using narcotics (acupuncture treatment can strengthen the effect of the narcotics).
- People with diminished mental capability who cannot give appropriate feedback on the effects of treatment.
- People prone to increased bleeding (hemophiliacs, persons on long-term steroid or blood thinning medications).

People with a needle phobia would better tolerate acupressure as a treatment choice. (See the NIH Consensus statement at *www.odp.od.nih.gov/consensus/cons/107/107_statement.htm*)

THERAPEUTIC MASSAGE

Therapeutic massage is a technique in which the soft tissue of the body (skin, muscle, tendons, etc.) is manipulated through touch. Practitioners use their hands, forearms, or elbows to apply pressure to specific areas during therapeutic massage. The primary difference between the many kinds of therapeutic massage in use today has to do with how hard, and in what way the soft tissue is manipulated. Shop around until you find the technique you best tolerate and like. Therapeutic massage is typically used along with physical therapy and chiropractic adjustments to reduce pain, improve movement, and restore function.

Clinical studies have found that therapeutic massage has both psychological and emotional effects on the body. Manipulation and massage of tight muscles relaxes them. This relaxation means that you will be able to get around with less pain. Massage increases circulation to the affected area, reduces inflammation, and aids in the healing of injured tissues. In addition, people often report a decrease of stress and anxiety during massage, which makes for an improved sense of well-being.

Therapeutic massage is performed by a licensed, trained individual in both clinical and home settings. Treatment sessions typically last 30 to 60 minutes, and the use of superficial heat prior to treatment is common. Traditional health insurance plans often cover therapeutic massage if it's ordered by a healthcare provider for a specific injury or disease process, and if treatment is delivered within a clinic setting.

Persons suffering from a recent injury with edema, bruising, and acute inflammation should not have therapeutic massage performed on the affected area. Persons with recent surgeries, circulatory problems, or impaired sensation should consult with their healthcare provider prior to starting treatment.

A person being treated with therapeutic massage must be able to relax and tolerate another person's touch. Only then can the treatment work. That's why people with skin hypersensitivity or contact phobia are not good candidates for therapeutic massage. Some cultures and religions restrict bodily touch or limit treatment by gender, so these facts must be considered prior to initiating therapeutic massage.

For further information, see (*www.ncbtmb.com/consumers_guide.htm.*)

HERBAL MEDICINES AND SUPPLEMENTS

Long before the corner drugstore existed, ancient healers used plants in the treatment of illness and pain. These plants, referred to as medicinal herbs, initially grew in the wild, but they were later cultivated to insure adequate supply. Healers verbally passed down their knowledge from generation to generation, but the spread of this knowledge outside individual cultures was limited by language, cultural practices, and geographical differences.

With the rise of traditional medicine, many cultures turned from the herbal practices of their ancestors. In the past 30 years, however, interest in using "natural" substances in the treatment of health has grown to the point that there are hundreds of medicinal herbs available today.

Supplements are usually vitamins, minerals, or other additives taken orally to meet the daily requirements for optimal health. Many people rely on supplements to "fill the gaps" of an unbalanced diet, or to insure adequate levels of substances that are naturally produced within the body.

Buy both medicinal herbs and supplements from a reliable

source. Quality and standardization of dosage can vary from brand to brand. Before using medicinal herbs or supplements, it's a good idea to consult with your healthcare provider, because herbs can interfere with some prescription medications.

The following overview of medicinal herbs and supplements will be confined to those used specifically for the treatment of pain:

Feverfew

Feverfew *(tanacetum parthenium)*: The leaves of this plant, a member of the daisy family, are used in the treatment of migraine headaches, arthritis, and other inflammatory diseases. Feverfew inhibits bodily changes that cause swelling, and it also ensures adequate circulation.

Feverfew can be taken orally in capsule form, applied topically in an ointment form, or by chewing its leaves. A typical dosage is one 100 mg tablet by mouth daily. Rare cases of toxicity have been reported with overuse, and mouth ulcers or irritation have been reported with chewing of the leaves.

Feverfew stimulates uterine contractions and should not be taken by pregnant/nursing women. People prone to increased bleeding (hemophiliacs and people using steroids or blood-thinning medications) should consult their healthcare provider before using Feverfew.

Capsaicin

Capsaicin *(capsicum annuum)*: This plant is a member of the red pepper family, and its pods are used in the treatment of arthritic pain and diabetic neuropathy/nerve pain. While capsaicin can be taken orally in capsule form, it is more commonly used in ointment form and is applied topically to the affected area. Clinical studies indicate that capsaicin blocks the ability of nerves to generate pain signals, thereby decreasing the level of perceived pain. A typical dosage is the application of between 0.025 percent and 0.075 percent.

Rare side effects include skin allergy to the ointment, and initial use of capsaicin can cause a feeling of strong, unpleasant burning to the treatment area (although this feeling tends to lessen with repeated use). Care must be taken to avoid getting capsaicin into the eye or nose areas. Capsaicin is a good choice for the treatment of specific, localized pain like shingles, diabetic neuropathic pain, and arthritis.

Willow bark

The bark of the willow tree (*salix alba*) has been called "nature's aspirin." It contains salicin, a natural compound that is chemically produced in laboratories as acetylsalicyclic acid, or bottled aspirin. Willow bark can be used as much as aspirin is for temporarily reducing pain, fever, and inflammation. Willow bark has the advantage of not causing the side effects of aspirin (stomach upset and decreased clotting ability). Willow bark is taken either orally in capsule form or brewed in tea form, although the tea can be very bitter tasting. A typical dosage is one 40 mg tablet, two to three times a day.

Persons who are prone to increased bleeding (hemophiliacs and people on steroid, or blood thinning medication) and those with disease processes that may be sensitive to aspirin (gout, asthma, diabetes, liver, or kidney dysfunction) should consult their healthcare provider prior to use. Persons taking prescription diuretics ("water pills"), high blood pressure medication, or an anti-inflammatory medication (like Advil or Motrin) should not use willow bark. To eliminate the risk of contracting Reye's syndrome, children under the age of 16 should never use willow bark.

St. John's Wort

St. John's Wort *(hypericum perforatum):* This plant has been used in the treatment of depression since the ancient Greeks and Hippocrates. It can also be used in the treatment of nerve pain and neuropathy often associated with diabetes or circulatory problems. The flower is dried and taken orally either in capsule form or brewed in a tea and can also be applied topically in ointment form.

One theory about how St. John's Wort works to decrease pain is that the active component, *hypericum,* promotes a greater sense of well-being, and may also reduce perceived levels of pain. Clinical studies are currently under way to better understand St. John's Wort and its healing properties. Rare side effects to St. John's Wort include sensitivity to the sun in fair-skinned people. Pregnant/nursing women and persons using prescription anti-depressant medications and should not use St. John's Wort.

If you are taking prescription medicines, consult with your doctor before taking this herb. Further, if you are to have surgery, stop taking St. John's Wort two weeks before. It can interact adversely with anesthesia and can cause blood pressure problems.

Glucosamine

This over-the-counter supplement is often used in the treatment of arthritis and joint pain. Glucosamine is a naturally produced substance within the body that maintains the ability of cartilage to act as "shock absorbers" for the joints. As a person ages, the body does not produce as much glucosamine and joint cartilage begins to deteriorate, causing pain and limited movement.

Clinical studies show that the use of supplemental glucosamine can slow the rate of deterioration of joint cartilage and reduce the effects of arthritis. Glucosamine can be taken in liquid or capsule form, and there are no known contraindications to use. A typical dosage is 1500 mg daily.

Chondrotin

Chondrotin: This over-the-counter supplement is often sold combined with glucosamine for the treatment of arthritis and joint pain. Clinical studies of chondrotin have shown no clinical benefits in its use and therefore use of chondrotin as a stand-alone supplement is not recommended.

Magnetic Therapy

This therapy is often recommended for pain treatment. Currently, scientific research does not show that magnets are an effective treatment. Clinical trials with larger numbers of people are needed to prove whether magnetic therapy is beneficial. Follow the reports on the web at *www.nccam.nih.gov/health/magnet/magnet.htm.*

Pain Matters

CAM is making its way into the mainstream even as scientific studies continue to seek greater understanding of individual therapies. In order to prevent potential harm or side effects, always check with your health care provider before beginning one of these therapies.

CHAPTER 13

Balancing Body, Soul, and Spirit

Jabez was more honorable than his brothers. His mother had named him Jabez, saying, "I gave birth to him in pain." Jabez cried out to the God of Israel, "Oh, that you would bless me and enlarge my territory! Let your hand be with me, and keep me from harm so that I will be free from pain." And God granted his request.

— 1 CHRON. 4:9–10

You can help manage your pain by eating a healthy diet, sleeping eight hours a night, getting proper exercise, and resting as needed during the day. You can also help yourself by pursuing hobbies you enjoy. Work itself can be therapy because it occupies your mind and reduces pain. Having a strong spiritual life can also benefit your health and well-being, and help you manage your pain, as many studies have shown.

Let's take a look now at diet, and the simplest way to begin is to look at the Healthy Diet Pyramid.

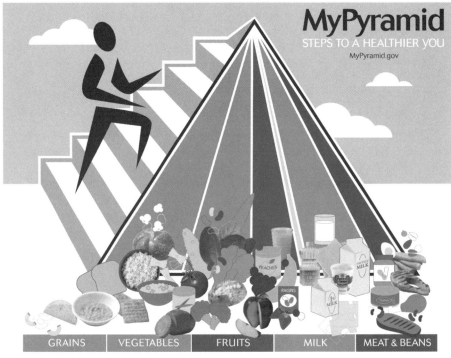

MyPyramid
STEPS TO A HEALTHIER YOU
MyPyramid.gov

GRAINS	VEGETABLES	FRUITS	MILK	MEAT & BEANS

GRAINS Make half your grains whole	**VEGETABLES** Vary your veggies	**FRUITS** Focus on fruits	**MILK** Get your calcium-rich foods	**MEAT & BEANS** Go lean with protein
Eat at least 3 oz. of whole-grain cereals, breads, crackers, rice, or pasta every day 1 oz. is about 1 slice of bread, about 1 cup of breakfast cereal, or ½ cup of cooked rice, cereal, or pasta	Eat more dark-green veggies like broccoli, spinach, and other dark leafy greens Eat more orange vegetables like carrots and sweetpotatoes Eat more dry beans and peas like pinto beans, kidney beans, and lentils	Eat a variety of fruit Choose fresh, frozen, canned, or dried fruit Go easy on fruit juices	Go low-fat or fat-free when you choose milk, yogurt, and other milk products If you don't or can't consume milk, choose lactose-free products or other calcium sources such as fortified foods and beverages	Choose low-fat or lean meats and poultry Bake it, broil it, or grill it Vary your protein routine — choose more fish, beans, peas, nuts, and seeds

For a 2,000-calorie diet, you need the amounts below from each food group. To find the amounts that are right for you, go to MyPyramid.gov.

Eat 6 oz. every day	Eat 2½ cups every day	Eat 2 cups every day	Get 3 cups every day; for kids aged 2 to 8, it's 2	Eat 5½ oz. every day

Find your balance between food and physical activity
- Be sure to stay within your daily calorie needs.
- Be physically active for at least 30 minutes most days of the week.
- About 60 minutes a day of physical activity may be needed to prevent weight gain.
- For sustaining weight loss, at least 60 to 90 minutes a day of physical activity may be required.
- Children and teenagers should be physically active for 60 minutes every day, or most days.

Know the limits on fats, sugars, and salt (sodium)
- Make most of your fat sources from fish, nuts, and vegetable oils.
- Limit solid fats like butter, stick margarine, shortening, and lard, as well as foods that contain these.
- Check the Nutrition Facts label to keep saturated fats, trans fats, and sodium low.
- Choose food and beverages low in added sugars. Added sugars contribute calories with few, if any, nutrients.

The foundation of the Healthy Eating Pyramid is daily exercise and weight control. Keeping a healthy weight, as the Healthy Weight Pyramid indicates, depends on knowing how much of each food group your body needs daily.

Whole Grain Foods (at most meals)

The body uses carbohydrates for energy. When you take in more carbohydrates than the body can use, these are stored as body fat. The latest diet fad is to minimize carbohydrates and make up the difference with protein and fats from meat and dairy foods. Such a diet can cause weight loss, but it is not balanced nutrition. Carefully selecting your sources of carbohydrates and keeping the proper balance among the food groups should be your goal.

The best sources of carbohydrates are whole grains such as oatmeal, whole-wheat bread, and brown rice. They deliver the outer (bran) and inner (germ) layers, along with energy-rich starch. A special advantage of whole grains is that the body can't digest them as quickly as it can highly processed carbohydrates such as white flour. This keeps blood sugar and insulin levels from rising, then

The best sources of carbohydrates are whole grains such as oatmeal, whole-wheat bread, and brown rice.

falling, too quickly. Better control of blood sugar and insulin can keep hunger at bay, and may prevent the development of type 2 diabetes. Bran is an excellent source of carbohydrates because it helps keep your bowel movements regular and prevents constipation. Bran also helps prevent colon cancer.

Plant Oils

Good sources of healthy unsaturated fats include olive, canola, soy, corn, sunflower, peanut, and other vegetable oils, as well as fatty fish, such as salmon. These healthy fats, when eaten in place of highly processed carbohydrates, not only improve cholesterol levels but can also protect the heart from sudden and potentially deadly rhythm problems. These oils help keep the body's clotting system in check so clots in the circulation to the brain (stroke) and heart (heart attack) are prevented.

Vegetables (in abundance) and Fruits (2 to 3 times)

A diet rich in fruits and vegetables can decrease the chances of having a heart attack or stroke; protect against a variety of cancers; lower blood pressure; help you avoid the painful intestinal ailment called diverticulitis; and guard against cataracts and macular degeneration, the major cause of vision loss among people over age 65.

Fish, Poultry, and Eggs (0 to 2 times)

These are important sources of protein. A wealth of research suggests that eating fish can reduce the risk of heart disease. Chicken and turkey are also good sources of protein and can be low in saturated fat. They should be baked or broiled, not fried. Eggs are also a good source of protein and vitamins.

Nuts and Legumes (1 to 3 times)

Many kinds of nuts contain healthy fats, and packages of some varieties (almonds, walnuts, pecans, peanuts, hazelnuts, and pistachios) can now even carry a label saying they're good for your heart. Nuts and legumes are excellent sources of protein, fiber, vitamins, and minerals. Legumes include black beans, navy beans, garbanzos, and other beans that are usually sold dried and canned.

Dairy or Calcium Supplement (1 to 2 times)

Building bone and keeping it strong takes calcium, vitamin D, exercise, sunlight, and a whole lot more. For Americans, dairy products have traditionally been the main source of calcium. But there are healthier sources of calcium other than milk and cheese, which can contain a lot of saturated fat. Three glasses of whole milk, for example, contains as much saturated fat as thirteen strips of cooked bacon. If you enjoy dairy foods, try to stick with no-fat or low-fat products. If you don't like dairy products, calcium supplements offer an easy and inexpensive way to get your daily calcium.

Red Meat and Butter (Use Sparingly)

These sit at the top (and narrowest part) of the Healthy Eating Pyramid because they contain lots of saturated fat. If you eat red meat every day, switching to fish or chicken several times a week can improve your cholesterol levels. So can switching from butter to olive oil.

White Rice, White Bread, Potatoes, Pasta, and Sweets with Refined Sugar (Use Sparingly)

They can cause fast increases in blood sugar that can lead to weight gain, diabetes, heart disease, and other chronic disorders. Whole-grain carbohydrates cause slower, steadier increases in blood sugar. Because the increases are slow, they don't overwhelm the body's ability to handle this much needed but potentially dangerous nutrient.

Multivitamin

A daily multivitamin that also contains a multimineral supplement offers a kind of nutritional backup. While it can't replace healthy eating or make up for unhealthy eating, it can fill in the nutrient holes that may sometimes affect even the most careful eaters. You don't need an expensive name brand or designer vitamin. A standard, store-brand, RDA-level one is fine. Look for one that meets the requirements of the USP (U.S. Pharmacopeia), an organization that sets standards for drugs and supplements.

Alcohol (in moderation)

Scores of studies suggest that having an alcoholic drink a day lowers the risk of heart disease. Moderation is clearly important, since alcohol has risks as well as benefits. For men, a good balance point is one to two drinks a day. For women, it's at most one drink a day.

KEEP AN EYE ON SERVINGS

Make sure the meals and snacks you eat contain items from several food groups. For example, a sandwich with whole wheat or rye bread may provide bread from the grains group, turkey from the meat and beans group, and cheese from the milk group. Choose a variety of foods for good nutrition. Individual foods in each group differ in their content of nutrients and other beneficial substances. By choosing a variety, you get *all* the nutrients and fiber you need. Variety can also help keep your meals interesting from day to day.

THERE ARE MANY HEALTHFUL EATING PATTERNS

Different people like different foods and different ways. Culture, family background, religion, moral beliefs, the cost and availability of food, life experiences, food intolerances, and allergies all affect people's food choices.

Make choices from each major group in the Pyramid, and combine them however you like. For example, if you like Mexican cuisine, you might choose tortillas from the grains group and beans from the meat and beans group, while people who eat Asian food might choose rice from the grains group and tofu from the meat and beans group.

If you usually avoid all foods from one or two of the food groups, be sure to get enough nutrients from other food groups. For example, if you choose not to eat dairy products because of intolerance to lactose or for other reasons, choose other foods that are good sources of calcium, and be sure to get enough vitamin D. Meat, fish, and poultry are major contributors of iron, zinc, and B vitamins in most American diets. If you choose to avoid all or most animal products, be sure to get enough iron, vitamin B12, calcium, and zinc from other sources. Vegetarian diets can meet recommended dietary allowances for nutrients.

For more information on nutrition, go to *www.nlm.nih.gov/medlineplus/nutrition.html*. You will find an interactive menu planner at *www.hin.nhlbi.nih.gov/menuplanner/menu.cgi*.

EXERCISE

In controlling pain, exercise is equally as important as diet. By keeping your muscles in tone, you can help yourself avoid or control muscle pain. All adults should get at least 30 minutes of moderate physical activity every day of the week. If you can't keep that schedule, three or four times a week is much better than none.

Exercise helps you to follow up on the weight loss you've achieved through your diet. For that purpose, more than 30 minutes of moderate physical activity daily is recommended. Over time, even a small decrease in the calories you eat and the physical activity you get each day can keep you from gaining weight or help you lose weight.

Exercise should be guided by your doctor or physical therapist. With their consultation, choose exercise that will not cause more pain or damage. Try to be more active throughout the day. Walk to nearby places where you would ordinarily ride, or take stairs for one or two flights instead of elevators.

But you should also get into a regular exercise routine. Regular walking, swimming, or sports activity can do the job. Weather needn't keep you from walking: You can walk in a closed shopping mall when the weather's bad. You may also want to get into an exercise routine in a gym. The YMCA and YWCA have exercise equipment and training for a reasonable fee, adjusted to your income.

Exercise gives you these benefits:

- Increases physical fitness.
- Helps build and maintain healthy bones, muscles, and joints.
- Builds endurance and muscular strength.
- Helps manage weight.
- Lowers risk factors for cardiovascular disease, colon cancer, and type 2 diabetes.
- Helps control blood pressure.
- Promotes psychological well-being and self-esteem.
- Reduces feelings of depression and anxiety.

SLEEP

Seven to eight hours of sleep each night helps the body to recover, helps muscles relax, and energy gets renewed. A good mattress with back support is important for those with back pain. To help you sleep through the night, take long-acting pain medication an hour before bedtime. Try not to exercise just before bedtime, and, after 6 P.M., avoid drinks that contain caffeine—such as coffee, tea, and sodas. Reading or relaxing with music before sleeptime helps many people fall asleep easier.

REST

Take rest breaks throughout the day. A short 10- to 15-minute nap can help you feel refreshed. Do not push your endurance limits. Exhaustion can aggravate your pain and your ability to cope with it. During the day, take time for a break from work pressures or stress: read a book, meditate, practice relaxation techniques, or listen to soothing music. Sometimes such activities can work even better than a nap in easing your body and mind.

WORK

Work can be therapeutic if it takes your mind off of the pain. The concentration work requires can help you forget your pain, or at least make it more tolerable. Avoid work that causes the injury or strain to increase. If the work you are doing increases injury or strain, you may have to think about changing jobs. Job training and vocational rehabilitation are available in many states. Your social worker or the state health service can tell you more about this.

If you are unable to work, you can volunteer your time and talents to your favorite community organization, hospital, house of worship, or school. As you help others, you will find your pain will be less.

FUN AS STRESS REDUCTION

> A *cheerful heart is good medicine, but a crushed spirit dries up the bones.*
>
> —PROVERBS 17:22 (NIV)

Continue to have fun with hobbies and activities you enjoy. Explore new hobbies if the old ones add more injury or stress. Plan a trip to somewhere you have always wanted to go.

Laughter is a good treatment. It helps take your mind off the pain and promotes health. Rent some funny movies to watch.

Share funny stories with friends and loved ones. Visit a comedy club and plan to laugh out loud.

Hobbies can also help. Many communities, high schools, and colleges offer evening classes in photography, painting, writing, travel, computers, gardening, and investing, among other subjects. Try out such new activities until you find one you enjoy and want to stick with. New hobbies will also bring new friends and serve as a fun distraction.

SPIRITUAL LIFE

A book called *Handbook of Religion and Health* by Harold George Koenig (Oxford University Press, 2000) draws on nearly 1,200 studies done on the effects of prayer on health. These studies show that religious people tend to live healthier lives. "They're less likely to smoke, to drink, [or] to drink and drive," Koenig says. In fact, people who pray tend to get sick less often, as separate studies conducted at Duke, Dartmouth, and Yale universities show. Some statistics from these studies are:

- Hospitalized people who never attended church have an average stay of three times longer than people who attended regularly.
- Heart patients were fourteen times more likely to die following surgery if they did not participate in a religion.
- Elderly people who never or rarely attended church had a stroke rate double that of people who attended regularly.
- In Israel, religious people had a 40 percent lower death rate from cardiovascular disease and cancer.

Koenig also finds that religious people "tend to become depressed less often. And when they *do* become depressed, they recover more quickly from depression. That has consequences for their physical health and the quality of their lives."

Several studies have demonstrated that your health can improve when others pray you for. This is called "intercessory prayer." Have your family, friends, and fellow church members pray for your recovery and your pain relief. But make your prayers reciprocal. Praying for the healing of others also will help your own pain become less.

SUPPORT

Many hospitals, health plans, churches, and communities have disease specific support groups. These may be posted at you clinic, the local newspaper, or community news. It is often helpful to network with people who face the same challenges you do.

Even more important than support groups is family support. Try not to let your pain isolate you from your family. Your immediate and extended family can be a source of strength and love that helps you cope. Spend time with your family doing activities that take your mind off of the pain by keeping you involved with others.

BALANCE

The art of life, whether you have pain or are pain-free, is to keep a balance between the things that claim your attention. People get in trouble when their lives are entirely built around one part of life. Start helping yourself by making a list of the five most important things in your life. A way to get going is to think about what you want people to remember you for: your life as a father, mother, husband, wife, teacher, volunteer, and so forth. Once you define your five priorities, write a mission statement for your life.

Your mission statement will probably include how and why you intend to give yourself to any of the five priorities you've named. This boils down to where you want to invest more of your time—family, hobby, exercise, your church, pain support group, etc.

Keep in mind that some of your priorities may include attention to yourself. To have power over pain you need enough rest, nutrition, family time, spiritual growth, hobbies, and fun.

To let pain run your life is to be seriously out of balance. All you need is the necessary knowledge that will put you, not your pain, back in charge.

Part Three

THE FUTURE OF PAIN TREATMENT

CHAPTER 14

Pain Challenges and Your Emotions

DEPRESSION, RACE, DISABILITY, AND DYING

Chronic pain can bring with it troubling emotional problems. To make matters worse, African Americans don't always get as good a pain management program as White people do, and that fact can obviously have its own emotional impact. Pain may also lead to disability and the depression that goes with it. In this chapter, we will take up these issues, as well as discuss the resources available to people who are dying—resources that can ensure that even through one's dying days, one can have the best possible quality of life.

DEPRESSION

Naturally, people who live with daily pain often experience mood problems, like anxiety/stress, insomnia, and severe depression. If chronic pain limits your ordinary activity, the problem can be even worse. We all need our independence, and when you can't do the things you used to do, you lose that independence.

We're beginning to know something about the psychology of chronic pain. Some studies suggest that chronic pain causes the same changes in brain function as those brought on by stress. The body reacts to stress by putting out stress hormones, such as adrenalin. Such hormones allow our hearts to beat faster and our responses to be quicker when we need to cope with, or flee from, danger. In times of chronic stress, such as stress brought on by chronic pain, our bodies continue to put out more stress hormones than usual, even though there is no sudden danger from which we must run.

Constant increased amounts of stress hormones affect our bodies in a variety of ways. It also can affect the mind. When you're stressed or in constant pain, your body doesn't produce enough serotonin. Serotonin helps to regulate several essential functions—such as sleep, mood, and anxiety. When you aren't getting enough serotonin, you're less able to fight depression, and, some investigators think, to deal with pain. That's why it's no surprise that people with chronic lower back pain are three to four times more likely to experience depression.

Depression can affect people with chronic pain in more than one way. Studies report that:

- People in pain who are depressed are more likely to rate their pain as severe than people who aren't depressed.
- When depression is accompanied by sleeplessness, you experience more pain and other physical symptoms, as well as depression.
- People with chronic pain and depression more frequently have suicidal thoughts, and attempts, than people with other chronic medical problems.

Chronically depressed people often don't know that they're depressed. That's why it's so important to be evaluated by your physician, who can determine whether depression is complicating your chronic pain situation. Treating the depression may help improve some of the pain symptoms. (It is urgent that you seek help if you have thoughts of helplessness or of harming yourself.)

Treatments for depression have also proved helpful in situations of chronic pain. Group programs, run by nurses with specialties in pain management, have been successful. Such programs work without medicines, emphasizing instead education and behavior changes. Studies have shown that such programs "reduce suffering and improve sense of well-being even for people who have experienced pain for many years."

Besides joining a support group, you may also want to see a therapist (psychologist or psychiatrist). Chronic pain sufferers continually experience the losses that go along with daily pain, as well as the accompanying physical changes. A therapist can often be helpful by encouraging you to look these losses in the face, and to learn to cope with your feelings about them.

If your physician recommends an antidepressant, understand that he or she is not telling you that your pain "is all in your head." The doctor is offering you an important tool for treating your pain. Many studies show that even in people who aren't depressed, chronic headaches, low back pain, or diabetes-related neuropathic (nerve ending injury) types of pain can be lessened through the use of antidepressants.

Commonly used antidepressants in pain treatment include older drugs, such as nortriptyline (Pamelor®) or amitriptyline (Elavil®). The best dose varies from person to person, and your physician will adjust your dosages to insure that you are taking the dosage that works best for you.

As to the power of the newer classes of antidepressants (SSRIs) to improve pain, the jury's still out. Some studies have shown improvement while others have not. There is some evidence that venlafaxine (Effexor®) is at least as effective as the older nortriptyline class, with fewer side effects. More work is needed to prove this.

FEAR AND ANXIETY

We have all experienced fear and anxiety at some time in our lives. In talking about fear, definitions make a good jumping-off place. Fear is defined in *www.yourdictionary.com* as follows:

1. a) A feeling of agitation and anxiety caused by the presence or imminence of danger; b) A state or condition marked by this feeling: living in fear.
2. A feeling of disquiet or apprehension: a fear of looking foolish.
3. Extreme reverence or awe, as toward a supreme power.
4. A reason for dread or apprehension: Being alone is my greatest fear.

Anxiety is defined in the same place as:

1. a) A state of uneasiness and apprehension, as about future uncertainties; b) A cause of anxiety: For some people, air travel is a real anxiety.
2. Psychiatry: A state of apprehension, uncertainty, and fear resulting from the anticipation of a realistic or fantasized threatening event or situation, often impairing physical and psychological functioning.
3. Eager, often agitated, desire: My anxiety to make a good impression.

Chronic pain causes fear and anxiety about our abilities to function and to be productive in our lives. We worry about the deterioration of our bodies and we worry about our future. We ask questions like:

"Do I have some dreadful disease that will harm me?"

"The doctors don't know what's wrong with me. Is there something they've missed?"

"How will I continue to function?"

Anxiety, bad enough in itself, when mixed with chronic pain, causes you to experience still more pain.

In children who have undergone repeated painful procedures, each repeat episode is associated with increased anxiety, as well as the reported intensity of the pain. In adults who have a liver biopsy, increased anxiety means the patient will require higher doses of pain medication for relief of pain. Data also suggests that in people with chronic headaches, anxiety connected with fear of pain made them require higher dosages of prescription pain medications.

The ability to feel "in control" of the situation can influence the degree of pain experienced. The more you know about what is causing your pain and how you can best control it, the less your anxiety and pain.

Because they know that anxiety makes the pain worse, doctors often prescribe anti-anxiety medications for people with chronic pain. Medications used to control anxiety include tranquilizers in the benzodiazepine class, antidepressants, and antihistamine medications with anti-anxiety actions.

The benzodiazepines include diazepam (Valium®), alprazolam (Xanax®), and lorazepam(Ativan®), among others. They are effective in calming anxiety, but, with regular use, can cause physical dependence. Hydroxyzine (Vistaril®), in the antihistamine family, has anti-anxiety effects without the posing dependence problems. Drowsiness is a possible side effect with either group. Buspirone (Buspar®), which is not a benzodiazepine, is specifically indicated for "generalized anxiety disorder."

As for non-medication treatments, those proven effective include:

- Counseling.
- Distraction.

- Relaxation exercises, like meditation.
- Music therapy.

Music can be a powerful part of your anti-pain program. Harp music has been shown to help decrease pain and anxiety in patients recovering from surgery in an Intensive Care Unit. Another study, done with patients who were about to have shock wave therapy to dissolve kidney stones, found that music, by itself, worked better to lower patients' anxiety than anti-anxiety medicine did. (For more on non-medication treatments, see Chapter 10.)

RACE AND PAIN

Study after study shows that if you're a "minority," you probably won't get as good a pain management program as a member of the "majority" population. It's the same picture, time after time, whether it happens in emergency rooms, hospitals, or cancer clinics.

We know something about why this happens. Most medical schools don't teach doctors how to deliver good pain therapy. But what complicates that fact is that in many areas of healthcare, there's little racial sensitivity and sometimes there's prejudice. The good news is that medical institutions *are* beginning to awaken to these issues. In some medical schools, at least, there are now courses in good pain management and in racial sensitivity. You've heard it too often already, but here it is again: Change takes time. In the meantime, you can lower your anxiety by insisting on good pain therapy. You might even want to bring this book with you, so as to better inform the doctor what good pain therapy is.

BECOME PROACTIVE AND BECOME AN ADVOCATE

The best way to be sure that you get the best possible treatment for pain is to know what that treatment should be, under the particular circumstances. After you've read this book, you will know more about pain management than many doctors in practice. So be assertive in asking questions about your treatment options, and why you think the doses may be too low. Know there is a chain of command in the clinics and hospitals. If your provider seems unwilling to give you the treatment you deserve, insist on talking with someone higher up the ladder. Once you and your provider have agreed on the best possible treatment plan, work with your provider to draw up a typed individual pain treatment guide that you can carry when you travel.

Besides knowing how to help yourself, you may also want to address the issue of pain management on a community level. Try to identify health care providers in your community willing to be champions for excellent and equal pain treatment for all. Work with them to have guidelines for pain management put in the emergency rooms (including the one you use), and in doctors' offices where pain treatment is common.

Some people want to go still farther. Why not:

- Offer to speak at medical programs, schools, and support groups.
- Write an article for your local newspaper.
- Talk to your TV news stations about a story on pain management.
- Raise funds for pain research by having a fund raiser, a march, a walk, or a run.
- Write your legislators in your state and in Congress about the need for pain management programs, research for better treatments and better professional education.

You'll find that nothing can better distract you from your pain than becoming an advocate for proper treatment of pain.

An excellent starting point is the "Take Action Now" button on the American Pain Foundation's website, *www.painfoundation.org.*

DISABILITY

The definition of disability in the Social Security law is strict. To be eligible for benefits, you must be unable to do any kind of substantial, gainful work because of a physical or mental impairment(s). The disability is expected either to last for at least twelve months or to end in death.

Even if your medical condition makes it impossible to do the work you performed in the past, Social Security requires that your age, education, and past work experience be considered in determining whether you can do other work. Only if the findings show that you can't perform other work do you become eligible for Social Security disability benefits.

You should be familiar with the process Social Security Administration uses to determine if you are disabled. It's a step-by-step process involving these five questions:

1. Are you working? If you are working and your earnings average more than $800 a month, you generally cannot be considered disabled.
2. Is your condition severe? Your impairments must interfere with basic work-related activities for your claim to be considered.
3. Is your condition found in the Social Security Administration's list of disabling impairments? If your condition is not on the list, the people doing the assessment must decide if it is of equal severity with impairment on the list. If it is, your claim is approved. If it is not, we go to the next step.

4. Can you do the work you did previously? If your condition is severe, but not at the same or equal severity as an impairment on the list, then Social Security people must determine if it prevents you from doing the work you did in the last 15 years. If it does not, your claim will be denied. If it does, your claim will be considered further.
5. Can you do any other type of work? If you cannot do the work you did in the last fifteen years, they will look to see if you can do any other type of work.

Answering that involves taking into consideration your:

- Age.
- Education.
- Past work experience.
- Transferable skills.
- Demands of various occupations as determined by the Department of Labor.

If you cannot do any other kind of work, your claim will be approved. If you can, your claim will be denied.

You may obtain a copy of *Disability Evaluation Under Social Security* ("The Blue Book") (5/02; SSA Publication No. 64-039), at *www.ssa.gov/disability/professionals/bluebook*. This document contains the medical criteria that SSA uses to determine disability. While it is intended primarily for physicians and other health professionals, it can be useful to you as you prepare to apply for disability.

If you believe that you meet the qualifications for Social Security disability benefits, see instructions for applying for disability benefits at *www.ssa.gov/disability.html*.

Or you can apply online for Disability benefits at *www.ssa.gov/applyforbenefits*.

HOSPICE AND PALLIATIVE CARE AT THE END OF LIFE

Dying can be accompanied by pain, as we all know. Such pain can be greatly relieved, or even eliminated, by the right kind of care. An especially strong resource for the dying person, and his or her loved ones, is Hospice, which specializes in compassionate, palliative care at the end of life. "Palliative" means to relieve without curing, and we all entitled to such care when the end of life is near.

Palliative care involves a team-oriented approach that includes:

- Expert medical care.
- Pain management.
- Emotional support.
- Spiritual support according to the patient's wishes.

Hospice also extends emotional and spiritual support to the family and loved ones.

For the most part, Hospice care is provided in the patient's home or in a home-like setting operated by a hospice program. In most states, Medicare, private health insurance, and Medicaid cover Hospice care for patients who meet the criteria.

The goal of palliative care is the best possible quality of life for patients and their families. Today, there are more and more specialists in hospitals who can ensure that dying people get good pain management as needed, not just in their last days but also early in the process. It is the goal of the team to keep you pain free and functional for as long as possible.

If you have a disease that causes pain and that will end your life, you are eligible for palliative pain management and Hospice care. You will have the choice and support to stay in your home or a home-like care house instead of in a hospital room. These programs offer support to you and your family, and treat patient and loved ones as people who, besides having a body, have a mind and spirit.

Ask your primary-care provider about local Hospice and palliative-care services, if you feel you need them. Minorities too rarely use these services. We hope that changes. Find out more about Hospice, a service that can bring true comfort to the dying person and the family.

Learn more at:

www.hospicenet.org
www.hospicefoundation.org
www.nhpco.org
www.hospicepatients.org

Pain Matters

- Depression and anxiety often accompany chronic pain, but they can be relieved both by your knowledge of your special condition and, if necessary, by medication.
- It is possible that you will not be given the best pain treatment because you are Black or Latino. If you encounter such a situation, your knowledge of what a good treatment program will be should help persuade your doctor to provide the help you need.
- If your pain disables you, the Social Security Administration may offer you benefits.
- No one has to die frightened and in pain. Contact Hospice, who can provide you with their good services.

CHAPTER 15

Why Participate in a Clinical Trial?

He will wipe every tear from their eyes. There will be no more death or mourning or crying or pain, for the old order of things has passed away."

—REV. 21:4

Even as you read this, people across the country are working to find new medication and methods for treating pain, and to learn more about the diseases that cause pain. This research goes on in the form of "clinical trials," in which those new medications and methods are tested both for their effectiveness and their safety.

Patients who are a part of such studies do better than patients who do not. That is because the study provides expert medical care, the latest information, free lab studies, and free treatment. To find the latest research in a particular area, go to the Internet site, *www.ClinicalTrials.gov.* You can also find helpful information at all the different pain clinical trials by clicking the "Clinical Trials" button at the American Pain Foundation website, *www.painfoundation.org.* If your pain is related to a disease, you'll find information on clinical trials here. You may also contact your nearest medical school, university, or your primary-care provider to learn about research going on in your area.

PLACEBO EFFECT

Some trials will be designed to explore the power of the mind to strengthen and help heal the body. In such trials, some patients will be given the active medication being explored, but others will be given a placebo. A placebo is an inactive pill, liquid, or powder that provides no treatment value. The placebo effect means that up to 30,000 people out of 100 will get better or have less pain by taking the placebo rather than an effective medication. This is testimony to the power of the mind in healing.

AN INTRODUCTION TO CLINICAL TRIALS

Choosing to participate in a clinical trial is an important personal decision that most people don't want to make alone. Instead, they talk to their physician and to family members or friends before deciding. Once you have identified trials that might help you, contact the study research staff and ask questions about these trials. That way, you'll know that either decision you make will be a good decision. For a list of active trials going on in your area, see *www.clinicaltrials.gov*.

Here are some frequently asked questions and answers that will let you see in more detail what clinical trials are about.

What is a clinical trial?

A clinical trial is a research study to answer specific questions about vaccines, new therapies, or new ways of using known treatments. Clinical trials (also called medical research or research studies) are used to determine whether new drugs or treatments are both safe and effective. Carefully conducted clinical trials are the fastest and safest way to find treatments that work.

Why participate in a clinical trial?

By participating, you play a more active role in your health care by gaining access to new research treatments before they are widely available. At the same time, by playing a part in medical research, you help others to enjoy the benefits that medical research provides in the way of best medications and treatment.

Where do the ideas for trials come from?

Ideas for clinical trials usually come from researchers, who have already tested new therapies or procedures on animals and got promising results. Now they are ready for a human trial that will turn up more and more information about a new treatment, its risks, and its benefits.

Who sponsors clinical trials?

Clinical trials are sponsored, or funded, by a variety of organizations or individuals–such as physicians, medical institutions, foundations, voluntary groups, and pharmaceutical companies, as well as federal agencies such as the National Institutes of Health (NIH), and the Department of Defense (DOD). Trials can take place in a variety of locations, such as hospitals, universities, doctors' offices, or community clinics.

What is a protocol?

A protocol is a study plan on which all clinical trials are based. The plan is carefully designed to safeguard the health of the participants as well as to answer specific research questions. A protocol describes what types of people may participate in the trial; the schedule of tests, procedures, medications, and dosages; and the length of the study. While they are in a clinical trial, participants following a protocol are seen regularly by the research staff for the purpose of monitoring their health and determining the safety and effectiveness of their treatment.

What is a control or control group?

A control is the standard by which experimental observations are evaluated. In many clinical trials, one group of patients will be given an experimental drug or treatment, while the control group is given either a standard treatment for the illness or a placebo.

What are the different types of clinical trials?

- *Treatment trials* test new treatments, new combinations of drugs, or new approaches to surgery or radiation therapy.
- *Prevention trials* look for better ways to prevent disease in people who haven't had it, or for ways to prevent a disease from returning. These approaches may include medicines, vitamins, vaccines, minerals, or lifestyle changes.
- *Screening trials* test the best way to detect particular diseases or health conditions.
- *Quality of Life trials* (or Supportive Care trials) explore ways to improve the comfort and quality of life of people who must live with a chronic illness.

What are the phases of clinical trials?

Clinical trials are conducted in phases. The trials at each phase have a different purpose and help scientists answer different questions:

- In *Phase I trials*, researchers test for the first time a new drug or treatment in a small group of people (20 to 80) to evaluate its safety, determine a safe dosage range, and identify side effects.

- In *Phase II trials*, the drug or treatment is given to a larger group of people (100–300) in order to find out more about its safety and effectiveness.
- In *Phase III trials*, the study drug or treatment is given to large groups of people (1,000–3,000) to confirm its effectiveness, monitor side effects, compare it to commonly used treatments, and collect information that will allow the drug or treatment to be used safely.
- In *Phase IV trials*, post-marketing studies find additional information including the drug's risks, benefits, and optimal use.

What is an "expanded access" protocol?

Some patients don't qualify to participate in a test because of other health problems, age, or other factors. For patients who may benefit from the drug but don't qualify for the trials, FDA regulations enable manufacturers to provide for "expanded access" use of the drug.

As an example of expanded access, a Treatment IND (Investigational New Drug) protocol is a relatively unrestricted study. The primary intent of a treatment IND/protocol is to provide access to the new drug for people with a life-threatening or serious disease for which there is no good alternative treatment. A Treatment IND/protocol may also be used to generate additional information about the drug, especially its safety.

You can fall under an expanded access protocol only if clinical investigators are actively studying the new treatment in well-controlled studies, or if all studies have been completed. There must be evidence that the drug may be an effective treatment in patients like those to be treated under the protocol. The drug cannot expose patients to unreasonable risks as measured against the severity of the disease to be treated.

To locate an expanded access program, see *www.fda.gov/fdac/special/newdrug/speeding.html*.

PARTICIPATION IN CLINICAL TRIALS

If you are considering participating in a clinical trial, the following frequently asked questions would help you understand the role of the participant in clinical trials. For a list of active trials see *www.clinicaltrials.gov*.

Who can participate in a clinical trial?

All clinical trials have guidelines about who can participate. The factors that allow someone to participate in a clinical trial are called "inclusion criteria," and those that disallow someone from participating are called "exclusion criteria." These criteria are based on such factors as age, gender, the type and stage of a disease, previous treatment history, and other medical conditions.

Some research studies seek participants with illnesses or conditions to be studied in the trial, while others need healthy participants. So whether or not you are included in a trial hasn't anything to do with you personally. Rather, the criteria are designed to identify appropriate participants and keep them safe, as well as to help researchers find answers to the questions they plan to study.

What happens during a clinical trial?

The trial team includes doctors and nurses as well as social workers and other healthcare professionals. They check the health of the participant at the beginning of the trial, give specific instructions for participating in the trial, monitor the participant carefully during the trial, and stay in touch after the trial is completed.

Some clinical trials involve more tests and doctor visits than the participant would normally have for an illness or condition. For all types of trials, the participant works with a research team. Frequent contact with the research staff gives you the best likelihood of a good outcome.

What is informed consent?

Informed consent means that before you decide whether or not to participate in a clinical trial, you've learned the key facts about it. It is also means that the patient will be given further information during each stage of the trial.

To help you decide whether or not to participate, the doctors and nurses involved in the trial explain it in detail. If your native language isn't English, a translator can be provided. It is the researcher's responsibility to explain it in a way that you understand it.

Once you have understood the explanation, you'll be given an *informed consent document* that includes details about the study, such as its purpose, duration, required procedures, and key contacts. Risks and potential benefits are also explained in the document. Having taken all that in, you're ready to decide whether to sign the document. Informed consent is not a contract, and the participant may withdraw from the trial at any time.

How do I best prepare for the meeting with the research coordinator or doctor?

- Plan ahead and write down the questions you want to ask.
- Ask a friend or relative to come along for support and to hear the responses to your questions. Your friend may want to take notes.

- Bring a tape recorder to record the discussion to replay later.

What are some key issues I should discuss with the trial team?

The team will want you to know as much as possible about the clinical trial and feel comfortable asking the members of the health care team questions. You'll want to know what care you're provided while the trial goes on, and what part, if any, of the trial treatment you will have to pay for.

The following questions are the kinds of questions you'll want answers to. (Some of the answers to these questions are found in the informed consent document.)

- What is the purpose of the study?
- Who is going to be in the study?
- Why do researchers believe the new treatment being tested may be effective? Has it been tested before?
- What kinds of tests and treatments are involved?
- How do the possible risks, side effects, and benefits in the study compare with those of my current treatment?
- How might this trial affect my daily life?
- How long will the trial last?
- Will hospitalization be required?
- Who will pay for the treatment?
- Will I be reimbursed for other expenses?
- What type of long-term follow up care is part of this study?
- How will I know that the treatment is working?
- Will results of the trials be provided to me?
- Who will be in charge of my care?

Does a participant continue to work with a primary-healthcare provider(PHC) while in a trial?

Yes. Clinical trials provide short-term treatments related to a designated illness or condition, but do not provide extended or complete primary health care. By having your PHC work with the research team, you ensure that other medications or treatments you may be on will not conflict with the protocol.

What are side effects and adverse reactions?

Side effects are any undesired effects of a drug or treatment. Such effects include headache, nausea, hair loss, skin irritation, or other physical problems. Experimental treatments must be evaluated for both immediate and long-term side effects.

What are the benefits and risks of participating in a clinical trial?

Today, most clinical trials are well-designed and well-executed. They offer and encourage and enable you to:

- Play an active role in your health care.
- Gain access to new research treatments before they are widely available.
- Obtain expert medical care at leading health care facilities during the trial.
- Help others by contributing to medical research.

Risks

There are also risks to clinical trials.

- There may be unpleasant, serious, or even life-threatening side effects to treatment.
- The treatment may not work on you.
- The protocol may require more of your time and attention than you can give.

How is the safety of the participant protected?

The ethical and legal codes that govern medical practice in general also apply to clinical trials. Most clinical research is federally regulated and monitored, with built-in safeguards to protect you throughout the course of the trial. The trial follows a carefully controlled protocol—a study plan that lays out, in detail, what the researchers will do in the study.

Your protection doesn't stop there. While the trial is going on, your team will report results at scientific meetings, publish interim findings in medical journals, and also report interim findings to various government agencies.

In addition, every clinical trial in the U.S. must be approved and monitored by an Institutional Review Board (IRB) to make sure the risks are as low as possible as measured against the disease itself. An IRB is an independent committee of physicians, statisticians, community advocates, and others who work to ensure that a clinical trial is ethical and that the rights of study participants are protected. By federal regulation, all institutions that conduct or support biomedical research involving humans must have an IRB that initially approves and periodically reviews the research.

The bottom line is that your clinical plan, for as long as the trial lasts, is being reviewed not only by the team, but also by experts from around the country.

Can a participant leave a clinical trial after it has begun?

Yes. A participant can leave a clinical trial at any time. All that's required of you is to let the research team know you are leaving, and the reasons why.

Pain Matters

People, and especially minorities, sometimes avoid clinical trials because they fear they will be "experimented on." In fact, doctors and clinics that conduct clinical trials are usually the best in their field, and can offer you the best possible care with the latest treatment. Participating in a trial will lower your costs and provide you with services you might otherwise not have been able to get. Check out the facts about clinical trials that could help you, and make an informed decision.

CHAPTER 16

Summing Up

At this point, you can give yourself a pat on the back. By reading *Overcoming Pain*, you've learned a lot about the causes of pain and the treatments for it. You also have learned these basic facts:

- Pain is your body's early warning system, letting you know of injury or trouble.
- Pain signals can go awry and cause loss of function, sleep, occupation, and enjoyment of life.
- Chronic pain can lead to depression, insomnia, and inability to work. It can cost a great deal of money and time.

Such information prepares you to avoid the potentially crippling effect of chronic pain and makes you an educated consumer What you've learned in *Overcoming Pain* falls under the following headings:

- The causes and types of pain, and the best ways to manage them.
- The range of medicines that treat only one type or cause of pain (for example, the triptans, in migraine headaches), along with the medicines that help treat all types of pain.

- Non-medical treatments that may help you.
- The many types of doctors, therapists, clinics, and professionals available to help you.
- The various blood tests, X-rays, and scans doctors use to diagnose the exact cause of your pain, in order to provide the best treatment.
- The pain scales that help track how well your pain treatment is working.
- Why you may want to keep your own daily pain diary, to be shared with your healthcare provider to help ensure you the best possible care.
- The importance of keeping track of your mood, periods of pain and relief from pain, ability to function, and any side effects your medication may be causing.

We also want you to recognize the many non-medication treatments that can help in your battle. Such treatments help you get your mind off the pain and on to life's other important issues and enjoyments. Also helpful are good diet, exercise, and sufficient sleep.

Finally, another kind of knowledge you've gained is about why it's important to become a vocal advocate of quality pain treatment. Pain is usually undertreated in emergency rooms and clinics in America, especially if you are a Black or Latino. We've shown you how to join others in advocacy of the best possible pain management and care. And you're joined in your advocacy by a growing number of physicians who specialize in pain management, and of good pain clinics staffed by trained experts in pain.

No one wants to live with chronic pain. But, if you must, there are better and worse ways to deal with your problem. Millions of people have learned to face their pain and the fact that they may always have to cope with it. But that's what they do—they cope. They refuse to let pain rule their lives.

You, too, are ready to cope with what you can't change. By balancing the condition of the body against the things you want to do, you will learn to keep focused on what's most important to you. Feeding your spirit is an excellent way to get your priorities straight. Many people who struggle with chronic pain find that becoming part of a religious or spiritual community promotes healing and healthy living.

Shalom. Be at peace and in safety, be prosperous and happy, be in health, be whole and be well.

Part Four

FUTHER RESOURCES

Pain Assessment Tools

---

1. PAIN INVENTORY (SHORT FORM)

Here is a form for you to fill out before you go to your doctor or primary-care provider:

Date:_____ /_____ /_____

Time: _____

Name: _____
      Last   First   Middle Initial

1) Throughout our lives, most of us have had pain from time to time (such as minor headaches, sprains, and toothaches). Have you had pain other than these everyday kinds of pain today?

    1. yes   2. no

2) On the diagram, shade in the areas where you feel pain. Put an X on the area that hurts the most.

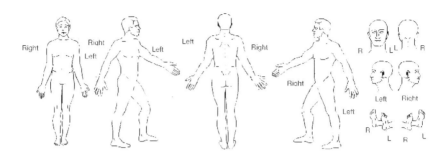

3) Please rate your pain by circling the one number that best describes your pain at its **WORST** in the past 24 hours.

0	1	2	3	4	5	6	7	8	9	10

No
pain

Pain as bad as
you can imagine

4) Please rate your pain by circling the one number that best describes your pain at its **LEAST** in the past 24 hours.

0	1	2	3	4	5	6	7	8	9	10

No
pain

Pain as bad as
you can imagine

5) Please rate your pain by circling the one number that best describes your pain on **AVERAGE**.

```
0   1   2   3   4   5   6   7   8   9   10
|                                       |
No                                      Pain as bad as
pain                                    you can imagine
```

6) Please rate your pain by circling the one number that tells how much pain you have **RIGHT NOW**.

```
0   1   2   3   4   5   6   7   8   9   10
|                                       |
No                                      Pain as bad as
pain                                    you can imagine
```

7) What treatments or medications are you receiving for your pain?

_____

_____

8) In the past 24 hours, how much **RELIEF** have pain treatments or medications provided? Please circle the one percentage that most shows how much.

```
0%  10%  20%  30%  40%  50%  60%  70%  80%  90%  100%
|                                                   |
No                                                  Complete
relief                                              relief
```

9) Circle the one number that describes how, during the past 24 hours, **PAIN HAS INTERFERED** with your:

A. General Activity

0	1	2	3	4	5	6	7	8	9	10

Does not
interfere

Completely
interferes

B. Mood

0	1	2	3	4	5	6	7	8	9	10

Does not
interfere

Completely
interferes

C. Walking ability

0	1	2	3	4	5	6	7	8	9	10

Does not
interfere

Completely
interferes

D. Normal work (includes both work outside the home and housework)

0	1	2	3	4	5	6	7	8	9	10

Does not
interfere

Completely
interferes

E. Relations with other people

0	1	2	3	4	5	6	7	8	9	10

Does not
interfere

Completely
interferes

F. Sleep

0	1	2	3	4	5	6	7	8	9	10

Does not
interfere

Completely
interferes

G. Enjoyment of life

0	1	2	3	4	5	6	7	8	9	10

Does not
interfere

Completely
interferes

Source: Pain Research Group, Department of Neurology, University of Wisconsin-Madison. Used with permission.

Note: May be duplicated and used in clinical practice.

2. INITIAL PAIN ASSESSMENT TOOL

Date:_____ /_____ /_____

Patient's name:_____ Age:_____ Room:_____

Diagnosis:_____

Physician:_____ Nurse:_____

I. *Location:* Patient or nurse marks drawing

II. *Intensity:* Patient rates the pain. Scale used: _____

  Present:_____

  Worst pain gets:_____

  Best pain gets:_____

  Acceptable level of pain:_____

III. *Quality:* (Use patient's own words, e.g., prick, ache, burn, throb, pull, sharp) _____

  _____

IV. *Onset, duration, variations, rhythms:*_____

V. *Manner of expressing pain:*_____

VI. *What relieves the pain?*_____

VII. *What causes or increases the pain?*_____

_____

VIII. *Effects of pain:*
(Note decreased function, decreased quality of life.)

Accompanying symptoms (e.g., nausea)_____

Sleep_____

Appetite_____

Physical activity_____

Relationship with others (e.g., irritability)_____

Emotions (e.g., anger, suicidal, crying)_____

Concentration_____

Other_____

_____

IX. *Other comments:*_____

_____

X. *Plan:*_____

_____

Source: McCaffery and Beebe, 1989. Used with permission.
Note: May be duplicated and used in clinical practice.

3. DAILY PAIN DIARY

Copy this form (make multiples or copy by hand), print it, and, please, fill it in three times a day. You'll find it to be a powerful communication tool when you next talk to your doctor.

Your doctor will want to know how well your pain medicine is working. You can help him or her come to conclusions by recording your pain level, three times a day for the next week, on the chart below. Also, indicate how pain has affected your daily activities, if at all, and by also recording side effects you believe may have been caused by your pain medicine. Record the date and time when they occurred, and what you did about them.

Circle the numbers below that best describe how pain has interfered with your daily functioning this past week.

(0 = Does not interfere   10 = Completely interferes.)

General Activity   0 1 2 3 4 5 6 7 8 9 10

Mood   0 1 2 3 4 5 6 7 8 9 10

Walking Ability   0 1 2 3 4 5 6 7 8 9 10

Normal Work Routine   0 1 2 3 4 5 6 7 8 9 10

Relations With Other People 0 1 2 3 4 5 6 7 8 9 10

Sleep   0 1 2 3 4 5 6 7 8 9 10

Enjoyment of Life   0 1 2 3 4 5 6 7 8 9 10

Ability to Concentrate   0 1 2 3 4 5 6 7 8 9 10

Appetite   0 1 2 3 4 5 6 7 8 9 10

Pain Diary for week of _____

Each morning, midday, and night, record pain level on a scale of 1 to 10.

	Day 1 Pain			Day 2 Pain			Day 3 Pain			Day 4 Pain			Day 5 Pain			Day 6 Pain			Day 7 Pain		
	Morning	Midday	Nighttime	Morning	Midday	Nighttime	Morning	Midday	Nighttime	Morning	Midday	Nighttime	Morning	Midday	Nighttime	Morning	Midday	Nighttime	Morning	Midday	Nighttime
Worst Pain 10																					
Imaginable 9																					
8																					
7																					
6																					
5																					
4																					
3																					
2																					
1																					
No Pain 0																					
Rescue Doses Needed																					
Current Regimen Dosage																					
Adjustments (if any)																					

Please list any side effects that you think may have been caused by your pain medicine.

Side Effects	When	Doctor's Instructions	What You Did About Them
_____	_____	_____	_____
_____	_____	_____	_____
_____	_____	_____	_____
_____	_____	_____	_____
_____	_____	_____	_____
_____	_____	_____	_____
_____	_____	_____	_____

4. WRITING DOWN YOUR MEDICAL HISTORY

Seventy percent of the time doctors diagnose on the basis of your medical history. Only you know the important details in that history. So it is very important that you put your medical history in order, including:

- Your own history in clear order.
- The histories of other members of your extended family.
- The pain (and other) medications you are taking.
- The specific pain problem that brought you to the doctor's office.
- Questions you want to ask.

Your coming in with notes is a big help to your doctor's caring for you. Nowadays, your doctor will have only a limited amount of time to diagnose your problem, prescribe a treatment, and educate you about the whole process.

You can further help the accuracy and speed of the process by doing the following:

- Arrive for your appointment on time, or even a little early.
- Be clear about the main symptom you want addressed.
- Be able to describe these aspects of your pain:
  - Location.
  - Quality.
  - Severity.
  - Timing.
  - What makes it better.
  - What makes it worse.

Write down all of your medicines, dosages, including health foods, supplements, vitamins, and over-the-counter medications.

You may want to arrange your notes with the help of two simple memory devices. The first is "A History," and that is just what it is—a way of organizing the information that makes up your medical history:

A—Allergies to medications, foods, or other.

H—Hospitalizations.

I— Illnesses, such as diabetes, asthma, high blood pressure, etc. **I** is also for *immunizations,* such as tetanus, flu, pneumococcal, hepatitis B, etc.

S— Surgeries.

T— Trauma, Major accidents and injuries.

O—Oral medications.

R— Reproductive history.

Y— Youth illnesses.

On a separate page, list diseases that members of your extended family have experienced (cancer, diabetes, heart disease, hypertension, anemia, arthritis. etc.) Mention any contact you may have had with relatives who have a contagious disease.

A second device that's helps you to organize your social and lifestyle issues is called "FLAMES" and it's useful in organizing your social history, which the doctor will also need. Before your first visit, write notes on the following:

F— Family, food.
L— Lifestyle.
A— Abuse of substances and of the body.
M—Marital or significant other relationships.
E—Employment.
S— Support systems, such as, home life, friends, family, religion, etc.

Finally, with the help of your primary-care doctor, write an emergency room plan. You may sometimes have to seek treatment after hours, or because you are having a pain that needs immediate medical response. In such cases, emergency-room treatment might be the fastest and best you can get under the circumstances. The plan should include the medications you take, with dosages, and the lab tests you may need.

An emergency room plan saves time and avoids hassle, both for you and the ER staff. If you always go to the same emergency department, you may want to give them a copy of your ER plan.

Resources

ON THE INTERNET

The Internet is a fast and efficient way to find out anything you need to know. If you don't have a computer at home, go to your public library, where someone will help you to get started.

The following U.S. government web sites guide you to answers to your questions, provide contacts to clinical trials, as well as information on drugs and important health care issues. (All the clinical trials discussed in these sites are also available at *www.ClinicalTrials.gov*)

National Institutes of Health.

The NIH Clinical Center in Bethesda, Maryland, is the research hospital of the National Institutes of Health (NIH). There, through clinical research, scientific discoveries in the laboratory are translated into new and better medical treatments and therapies for people.

The Clinical Center's website guides potential participants, their families and physicians in their decision whether to participating in a trial is the best way to treat their particular case.

If you have decided to participate in one of these trials, the NIH provides recruitment information for sick or healthy participants at *www.cc.nih.gov/ccc/prrc/info.html#patients*.

The National Cancer Institute

The National Cancer Institute (NCI) is the U.S. government's center for clinical trials on cancer. Big U.S. government agencies that conduct cancer research, such as DOD or VA, do so in partnership with NCI. On the Web: *www.nci.nih.gov*.

NCI provides information that helps you to understand cancer trials, types of cancer, finding trials, resources for researchers, most requested pages, and more: *www.cancer.gov/clinical_trials*.

NCI Clinical Trials Education Series provides publications for individuals and health care professionals to help them understand clinical trials. These publications include self-paced workbooks, slide programs on CD-ROM, booklets, and videos: Learn about these at *www.oesi.nci.nih.gov/series/cted*.

The National Center for Complementary and Alternative Medicine at *www.altmed.nih.gov*.

The FDA Cancer Liaison Program, Office of Special Health Issues

This agency, with NCI, answers questions by participants, their families, and participant advocates about therapies for life-threatening diseases: *www.fda.gov/oashi/cancer/cancer.html*.

The National Institute of Mental Health (NIMH)

The NIMH provides "A Participant's Guide to Mental Health Clinical Research": *www.nimh.nih.gov/studies/clinres.cfm*.

The NIH Office of Extramural Research (OER), and the NIH Inter-Institute Bioethics Interest Group.

OER provides information on policies and regulations, Institutional Review Board resources, guidance for clinical investigators, research resources, and courses and tutorials on bioethical issues in human studies: *www.nih.gov/sigs/bioethics*.

The National Library of Medicine (NLM)

NLM has compiled a comprehensive bibliography from 1989 through November 1998, entitled "Ethical Issues in Research Involving Human Participants: *www.nlm.nih.gov/pubs/cbm/hum_ exp.html*.

HHS Office of Human Research Protection (OHRP)

OHRP provides a guide and training materials on regulations and procedures governing research with human subjects; includes a guidance document on financial relationships in clinical research: *www.ohrp.osophs.dhhs.gov/polasur.htm*.

The American Pain Foundation (AFP)

APF offers a wide selection of pain information. By clicking on one of several buttons, people can find out information or available treatments, clinical trials, pain management, patient advocacy, and a complete A-to-Z reference on pain. The APF website is *www.painfoundation.org*.

INFORMATION ON MEDICARE COVERAGE

Centers for Medicare and Medicaid Services (CMS) provide information on the recent (September 19, 2000) decision regarding Medicare payments for routine costs, and reasonable and necessary items in clReference e Coverage Policy-Clinical Trials at *www.medicaid.com/coverage/8d2.asp*.

Also read the quick Reference Guide at *www.medicaid.com/ medlearn/refctmed.asp*.

MEDLINEplus

The "Health Topics" section of the website has a web-based information service from the National Library of Medicine. "Health Topics" makes available reliable information about more than 550 diseases and conditions, as well as a link to clinical trials. It also includes an informative "Clinical Trials" health topic page, with some material in Spanish, and an interactive tutorial on clinical trials. *www.nlm.nih.gov/medlineplus/clinicaltrials.html*.

INFORMATION ON DRUGS

The Food and Drug Administration (FDA)

The FDA is the U.S. government agency responsible for ensuring the safety and effectiveness of all drugs. After a clinical trial, the FDA looks at the evidence to determine if a new drug or treatment is safe to approve as a marketable new product and if it is an improvement over the standard therapy.

FDA web sites provide valuable information to consumers on its activities in regulation and approval of drugs: *www.fda.gov*.

FDA also provides the following general information about newly approved prescription drugs:

- Information on how drugs are developed in the U.S.: "From Test Tube to Participant: New Drug Development in the U.S.":
  www.fda.gov/cder/about/whatwedo/testtube.pdf.
- Consumer information about drugs approved since 1998:
  www.fda.gov/cder/consumerinfo
- Information on products regulated by FDA:
  www.fda.gov/cder/drug/
- New and generic drug approvals since 1988:
  www.fda.gov/cder/approval/
- FAQs to CDER:
  www.fda.gov/cder/about/faq
- The FDA Electronic Orange Book, which gives current approved drug products:
  www.fda.gov/cder/ob

- MEDLINEplus Guide to over 9,000 prescription and over-the-counter medications: *www.nlm.nih.gov/medlineplus/druginformation.html*

DISEASE SPECIFIC RESOURCES

Angina—Chest Pain
American Heart Association: www.americanheart.org

Arthritis Pain
Arthritis Foundation: www.arthritis.org

Rheumatology
American College of Rheumatology: www.rheumatology.org

Cancer pain
City of Hope Pain/Palliative Care Resource Center (COHPPRC); City of Hope National Medical Center: www.cityofhope.org.
This is an excellent site for information about pain assessment, treatment, and specialized resources, such as sickle cell pain management. There are links to other pain related sites:

American Cancer Society: www.cancer.org

National Cancer Institute: www.nci.nih.gov

Wisconsin Cancer Pain Initiative (WCPI): *www.wisc.edu/wcpi*

Back and Neck Pain
Spine-Health.com: www.spine-health.com

Diabetes Pain
American Diabetes Association: www.diabetes.org

Headache Pain
National Headache Foundation: www.headaches.org

Hemophilia Pain
National Hemophilia Foundation: www.hemophilia.org/home.htm

HIV Pain
HIV Insight: www.hivinsite.ucsf.edu

Pelvic Pain
International Pelvic Pain Society: www.pelvicpain.org

Sickle Cell Pain
NIH Sickle Cell Center: www.rhofed.com/sickle
This site lists all federally funded centers, with e-mail addresses and locations.

Sickle Cell Disease Association of America: www.sicklecell disease.org
This site provides a state-by-state listing of member chapters where you can get sickle cell information, as well as local referrals.

Sickle Cell Information Center: www.SCInfo.org
This site offers a comprehensive information resource for patients, family members, health care providers and others seeking information about sickle cell disease and pain management.

GENERAL PAIN ORGANIZATIONS
American Pain Foundation: www.painfoundation.org.
A comprehensive site on pain that offers information on clinical trials, patient advocacy, treatment options, and more.

American Pain Society: www.ampainsoc.org

   A multidisciplinary organization of basic and clinical scientists, practicing clinicians, policy analysts, and others. Their mission is to advance pain-related research, education, treatment, and professional practice.

Partners Against Pain: www.partnersagainstpain.com.

StopPain.org at Beth Israel Medical Center: www.stoppain.org

National Foundation for the Treatment of Pain:
www.paincare.org

National Library of Medicine: www.nlm.nih.gov/medlineplus/

National Guideline Clearinghouse: at www.guideline.gov/index.asp

American Chronic Pain Association (ACPA): www.theacpa.org

Mayday Pain Center: www.painandhealth.org

National Pain Education Council Education Resource: www.
npecweb.org

   The American Pain Foundation website, at www.painfoundation.org, is an online resource for people with pain, and for their families, friends, caregivers, and the general public. This site is devoted to patient information and advocacy, and provides many links to additional resources. The APS web site will direct you to various resources for finding a pain specialist to treat your pain, and also to support groups and information.

World Wide Congress on Pain: www.pain.com
This is a comprehensive site about pain management with many links to other good websites.

HOW TO FIND PHYSICIAN PAIN SPECIALISTS

American Academy of Pain Management: www.aapainmanage.org

American Academy of Pain Medicine: www.painmed.org

American Society of Interventional Pain Physicians: www.asipp.org

Canadian Pain Society: www.medicine.dal.ca/cps

Center to Advance Palliative Care (CAPC): www.capcmssm.org

International Association for the Study of Pain: www.iasp-pain.org

Society for Pain Practice Management: www.sppm.org

American Society of Addiction Medicine: www.asam.org

PAIN IN CHILDREN

Pediatric Pain Sourcebook: www.dal.ca/~painsrc

University of Iowa College of Nursing—Pediatric Pain: www.nursing.uiowa.edu/sites/PedsPain

END OF LIFE PAIN

Medical College of Wisconsin Palliative Medicine Program: www.mcw.edu/pallmed

ADDITIONAL INTERNET RESOURCES

The Center to Advance Palliative Care (CAPC): www.capcmssm.org

International Association for the Study of Pain: www.iasp-pain.org

Mayday Pain Center: www.painandhealth.org

National Foundation for the Treatment of Pain: www.paincare.org

Pain.com: www.pain.com

National Library of Medicine: www.nlm.nih.gov/medlineplus

National Guideline Clearinghouse: www.guideline.gov/index.asp

Partners against Pain: www.partnersagainstpain.com

Society for Pain Practice Management: www.sppm.org

American Society of Addiction Medicine: www.asam.org

American Academy of Pain Management: www.aapainmanage.org

University of Iowa College of Nursing—Pediatric Pain: www.nursing.uiowa.edu/sites/PedsPain

Stop Pain: www.stoppain.org

Medical College of Wisconsin Palliative Medicine Program:
www.mcw.edu/pallmed

Wisconsin Cancer Pain Initiative (WCPI): www.wisc.edu/wcpi

American Pain Foundation 201 N. Charles St., Suite 710
Baltimore, MD 21201–4111; phone: 410–783–7292; fax:
410–385–1832: *www.painfoundation.org*

Basic Pain Assessment in Adults An On-Line Continuing
Education Home Study Course for Nursing and Pharmacy
Professionals, Diane Scheb, RN, MSN Acute Pain Program
Coordinator and Clinical Nurse Specialist Sarasota Memorial
Hospital, Sarasota, Florida; Chris Pasero, RN, MS Pain
Management Consultant Rocklin, California:
www.baxter.com/doctors/iv_therapies/education/index.html

National Pain Education Council Education Resource:
www.npecweb.org. Investigate the tools, services, and CME/CE
programs that the National Pain Education Council.

NHLBI is a part of the Federal Government's National Institutes
of Health.
　　National Heart, Lung, and Blood Institute: www.nhlbi.nih.gov

Sickle Cell Disease Scientific Research Group 6701 Rockledge
Drive, MSC 7950 Bethesda, MD 20892–7950; phone:
301–435–0055; fax 301–480–0868: *www.nhlbi.nih.gov*
　　This site lists all of the federally funded centers with email
addresses and locations.

Sickle Cell Disease Association of America, 200 Corporate Point #945, Culver City, CA 90230–7633; phone: 1–800–421–8453, 310–216–6363; fax: 310–215–3722: *www.sicklecelldisease.org/programs.htm*

A state-by-state listing of member chapters where you can obtain sickle cell information and local referrals is located on their website at:

Sickle Cell Information Center: www.SCInfo.org

This site is a comprehensive information resource for patients, family members, healthcare providers and others seeking information about sickle cell disease and pain management.

CLINICS

A current list of pain clinics is maintained at the Pain.com's wonderful website *www.pain.com/painclinics*

If you have a family doctor, let him or her refer you to a pain specialist if you feel your pain would be better managed by an expert. Many pain specialists will evaluate you, offer a plan, and provide treatments, then have you return to your regular doctor.

SUPPORT GROUPS

Many cities have patient support groups for specific diseases. Check with the specialty clinics in the city for the contacts and meeting times. Support groups help you by hearing the success and helpful tips from those who have the same pain and problems. It is a good way to share, network, raise funds for research, and obtain help. If there is not a support group in your area, you can be the beginning of one by getting together patients with the same problems. You can post your meeting location in the local clinics, hospitals, and newspaper.

PAIN ORGANIZATIONS AND WEB SITES

American Academy of Head, Neck and Facial Pain: phone: 800–322–8651: *www.aahnfp.org*

AAHNFP's focus is on the diagnosis and treatment of TMJ.

American Academy of Hospice and Palliative Medicine: *www.aahpm.org*

American Alliance of Cancer Pain Initiatives: www.aacpi.org

American Hospice Foundation: www.americanhospice.org

Americans For Better Care of the Dying: www.abcd-caring.org

American Academy of Orofacial Pain: 10 Joplin Court, Lafayette, CA 94549–1913; phone: 510–945–9298; fax: 510–945–9299: *www.aaup.org*

American Academy of Pain Management: Richard S. Weimer, Ph.D., Executive Director, 13947 Mono Way #A, Sonora, CA 95373; phone: 209–533–9744; fax: 209–533–9750: *www.aapainmanage.org*

American Academy of Pain Medicine: Jeffrey W. Engle CMP, Account Executive, 4700 West Lake Avenue, Glenview, IL 60025–1485, phone: 847–375–4731; fax: 847–375–4777: *www.painmed.org*

American Association for Chronic Fatigue Syndrome: *www.aacfs.org*

Promotes the stimulation, coordination, and exchange of ideas for CFS research.

American Back Pain Association: P.O. Box 135, Pasadena, MD 21222–0135; phone: 410–255–3633; fax: 410–255–7338.

 American Board of Pain Medicine: 4700 W. Lake Avenue, Glenview, IL 60025; phone: 847–375–4726; fax: 847–375–6326; email: info@abpm.org: *www.abpm.org/index.htm*.

American Chronic Pain Association: Penny Cowan, P.O. Box 850, Rocklin, CA 95677–0850; phone: 916–632–0922; fax: 916–632–3208; email: ACPA@pacbell.net: *www.theacpa.org*.

American College of Osteopathic Pain Management and Sclerotherapy: 107 Male Avenue, Silverside Heights, Wilmington, DE 19808; Phone: 301–792–9280: *www.acopms.com*

American Pain Foundation: 201 N. Charles Street, Suite 710, Baltimore, MD 21201–4111; Phone: 888–615–7246; Fax: 410–385–1832; email: info@painfoundation.org: *www.painfoundation.org*

 APF fills the need for a strong, credible, grassroots organization that provides information to people living with pain and the public about pain management, and mobilizes them effectively in support of full access to possible treatments and a fuller living experience.

American Pain Society: www.ampainsoc.org

 The American Pain Society is a multidisciplinary organization of basic and clinical scientists, practicing clinicians, policy analysts, and others. The mission of the American Pain Society is to advance pain-related research, education, and treatment.

American Podiatric Medical Association: www.apma.org/index.html.

 APMA's site provides information about foot health and foot pain.

American Society for Action on Pain: Skip Baker, P. O. Box 3046, Williamsburg, VA 23187; email: skipb@widomaker.com: *www.druglibrary.org/schaffer/asap/index/htm*

ASAP seeks adequate and ongoing opioid or narcotic pain medicine, for all Americans who suffer with chronic pain.

American Society of Interventional Pain Physicians: 2831 Lone Oak Road, Paducah, KY 42003; phone: 270–554-9412; fax: 270–554-8987: *www.asipp.org*

ASIPP's primary focus is the accessibility of treatment for pain patients.

American Society of Law, Medicine & Ethics: www.aslme.org

This site provided information of a project on legal constraints on access to effective pain relief which developed the model Pain Relief Act.

American Society of Pain Management Nurses: Dr. Belinda Puetz, Executive Director, 7794 Grove Drive, Pensacola, FL 32514; phone: 850–473–0233; fax: 850–484-8762; email: *aspmn@aol.com*

American Society of Regional Anesthesia: Denise Wedel, MD, Current President; P. O. Box 11086; Richmond, VA 23230–1086: *www.asra.com*

Back Pain Association of America: P. O. Box 135, Pasadena, MD 21122–0135; phone: 410–255–3633; fax: 410–255–7338; email: backpainassoc@fmsn.com

This organization provides free quarterly newsletters and support groups in U.S.

CFIDS Association of America: www.cfids.org
    This organization is dedicated to conquering chronic fatigue and immune dysfunction syndrome (CFIDS).

Education for Physicians on End-of-Life Care: www.epec.net

End-of-Life Nursing Education Consortium: www.aacn.nche.edu/elnec

End-of-Life Physician Education Resource Center: www.eperc.mcw.edu

End-of-Life Nursing Education Consortium: www.aacn.nche.edu/elnec

End-of-Life Physician Education Resource Center: www.eperc.mcw.edu

Hospice & Palliative Nurses Association: www.hpna.org

Hospice Foundation of America: www.hospicefoundation.org

Innovations in End-of-Life Care: www.edc.org/lastacts

International Pelvic Pain Society: 2006 Brookwood Medical Center Drive, Suite 402, Women's Medical Plaza, Birmingham, AL 35209; phone: 205–877–2950 or US 800–624-9676: *www.pelvicpain.org*
    The International Pelvic Pain Society was incorporated to allow physicians, psychologists, physical therapists and basic scientists to coordinate, collect and apply this growing body of information, and to serve as a forum for professional and public education.

International Association for the Study of Pain: 909 NE 43rd Street, Suite 306, Seattle, WA 98105–6020; phone: 206–547–6409; fax: 206–547–1703: *www.halcyon.com/iasp*

Interstitial Cystitis Association: 51 Monroe Street, Suite 1402, Rockville, MD 20850; Phone: 301–610–5300 or 800–HELP ICA; Fax: 301–610–5308; email: ICAmail@ichelp.org: www.ichelp.org

Founded in 1984, the Interstitial Cystitis Association (ICA) is a not-for-profit health organization dedicated to providing patient and physician educational information and programs, patient support, public awareness and, most importantly, research.

Intractable Pain Association: Forest Tennant, MD, 338 S. Glendora Avenue, West Covina, CA 91790; Phone: 800.624.4540

Last Acts: www.lastacts.org

Mayday Pain Project: www.painandhealth.org

National Hospice and Palliative Care Organization: www.nhpco.org

National Institute for Healthcare Research: www.nihr.org

National Chronic Pain Outreach Association: Michael Troyer— Director, P. O. Box 274, Millboro, VA 24460; Phone: 540–862–9437; Email: ncpoa@cfw.com

National Foundation for the Treatment of Pain: *www.paincare.org*

NFTP is a not-for-profit organization dedicated to providing support for patients who are suffering from intractable pain, and their families, and friends.

National Pain Foundation: P.O. Box 102605, Denver, CO 80250–2605; phone: 303–756–0889; email: aardrup@painconnection.org: *www.paincare.org*

NPF is a non-profit organization that provides online education for pain patients and their families—your source for information about pain disease, treatment options, and links to support groups.

National Vulvodynia Association: P. O. Box 4491, Silver Spring, MD 20914-4491; phone: 301–299–0775: *www.nva.org*

Neuropathy Association: 60 E. 42nd Street, Suite 942, New York, NY 10165; Phone: 212–692–0662: *www.neuropathy.org*

New England Pain Association: Stewart A. Hinckley, Executive Director, P. O. Box 11086, Richmond, VA 23230–1086; phone: 804-282–4011; fax: 804-282–0090

Pain Society of Oregon: 2852 Willamette St., PMB 158, Eugene, OR 97405; phone: (541) 954-7038; email: admin@painsociety.com: *www.painsociety.com*

PSO's focus is to improve members' knowledge and use of community pain treatment resources and methods.

Painfree International Charitable Foundation: Jennifer Chu, M.D., Department of Rehabilitation Medicine—Ground Floor, White Building, Hospital of the University of Pennsylvania, 3400 Spruce Street, Philadelphia, PA 19104; phone: (215) 662–3259: *www.painfree-international.org*

PICF was started by patients of Jennifer Chu, M.D., to support research, provide guidance for the causation, clinical course, prevention, diagnosis and treatment of muscle aches and pains as typified in myofascial pain and fibromyalgia.

National Heart, Lung, and Blood Institute: www.nhlbi.nih.gov
    NHLBI is a part of the federal government's National
Institutes of Health.

Sickle Cell Disease Scientific Research Group: 6701 Rockledge
Drive, MSC 7950, Bethesda, MD 20892–7950; phone
301–435–0055; fax 301–480–0868: *www.nhlbi.nih.gov*
    This site list all of the Federally funded centers with email
addresses and locations.

Sickle Cell Disease Association of America: 200 Corporate Point
#945, Culver City, CA 90230–7633; phone 1–800–421–8453 ,
310–216–6363; fax 310–215–3722: *www.sicklecelldisease.org*
programs.htm
    SCDAA's website provides a state-by-state listing of member
chapters where you can obtain sickle cell information and local
referrals.

Society for Pain Practice Management: Steven P. Waldman, MD,
JD—Executive Director, 11111 Nall, Suite 202, Leawood, KS
66211; phone: 913–491–6451; fax: 913–491–6453: *www.sppm.org*

Trigeminal Neuralgia Association: Claire W. Patterson, President,
P. O. Box 340, Barnegat Light, NJ 08006; phone: 609–361–1014;
fax: 609–361–0982; Email: tna@csionline.net:
www.tna-support.org

Vulvar Pain Foundation: P. O. Drawer 177, Graham, NC 27253;
phone: 910–226–0704; fax: 910–226–8518: *www.vulvarpain*
foundation.org

INTERNATIONAL ORGANIZATIONS

National Association for Healthy Backs (UK): www.backpain.org
   NAHB provides support, contact, and information services
for those with all back problems.

Canadian Pain Society: Joan Hoskins, 50 Driveway, Ottawa, ON
K2P 1E2; phone: 613–234-0812; fax: 613–234-9894:
www.medicine.dal.ca/cps
   A chapter of the International Association for the Study of Pain.

Egyptian Pain Society for Management of Pain:
www.pain-eg.org
   This organization was founded in 1982 and now has 420
members all over Egypt.

Fibromyalgia Association of British Columbia: P. O. Box 15455,
Vancouver, BC Canada V6B-5B2

Institute for the Study and Treatment of Pain: 5655 Cambie
Street, Lower Floor, Vancouver, BC, Canada V5Z 3A4; phone:
604-264-7867; fax: 604-264-7860: *www.istop.org*

International Spinal Injection Society: www.spinalinjection.com
   This association of physicians interested in the development,
implementation, and standardization of percutaneous techniques
for the precision diagnosis of spinal pain.

North American Chronic Pain Association of Canada:
www.chronicpaincanada.org
   This self-help organization dedicated to providing support to
people in chronic pain, and to giving assistance in living their
lives to the fullest.

Pain Research Institute: www.liv.ac.uk/pri

Pain World: www.painworld.zip.com.au
This organization's purpose is to provide a central place where chronic pain sufferers and family members can access information and facilities that might help them deal with this debilitating condition.

Scottish Network for Chronic Pain Research: Jennifer Hood; phone: 01786 466338 or 0131 554 8160; email: JHood@QMUC.ac.uk: *www.sncpr.org.uk*
SNCPR's site is designed to serve the needs of a broad range of groups or individuals.

University of Wisconsin Pain & Policy Studies Group: www.medsch.wisc.edu/painpolicy
A World Health Organization Collaborating Center.

Vulval Pain Society: PO Box 514, Slough, Berks SL1 2BP United Kingdom: *www.vul-pain.dircon.co.uk*

BOOKS

The Chronic Pain Solution: The Comprehensive, Step- By-Step Guide to Choosing the Best of Alternative and Conventional Medicine by James N., Md. Dillard, Leigh Ann Hirschman Bantam Doubleday Dell Pub; 1st edition (August 27, 2002)

The Chronic Pain Control Workbook: A Step-By-Step Guide for Coping With and Overcoming Pain by Ellen Mohr Catalano, Ph.D. Kimeron N. Hardin (Contributor), Shelby P. Tupper (Illustrator) New Harbinger Pubns; 2nd edition (August 1996)

Mayo Clinic on Chronic Pain by David W. Swanson (Editor), Jeffrey Rome Publisher: Kensington Pub Corp; 2nd edition (November 2002)

Managing Pain Before It Manages You, Revised Edition by Margaret Caudill (Author), Margaret A. Caudill Guilford Press; Revised edition (November 30, 2001)

Fibromyalgia and Chronic Myofascial Pain: A Survival Manual (2nd Edition) by Devin J. Starlanyl, Mary Ellen Copeland New Harbinger Pubns; 2nd edition (June 30, 2001) ISBN: 1572242388

Mayo Clinic on Arthritis by Gene G., Md. Hunder (Editor), Mayo Clinic, Gene G. Hunder Kensington Publishing Corp.; 1st edition (March 15, 1999)

Power over Pain by Eric M. Chevlen, MD and Wesley Smith, International Task Force, 2002, Steubenville, Ohio

The Truth about Chronic Pain by Arthur Rosenfeld, Basic Books 2003

GLOSSARY

acute pain. The result of an injury or potential injury to body tissues and irritation of pain-sensing nerve fibers at the site of local tissue damage. This type of pain is usually time-limited and occurs after trauma, surgery, or a disease process. Acute pain is generally thought to have the biological functions of alerting the individual to harm and preparing for the "fight-or-flight" response to danger.

addiction. Is defined as a primary, chronic disease with genetic, psychosocial, and environmental factors influencing its development and manifestations. Addiction involves a compulsive desire to use a drug despite continued harm. Addiction should be differentiated from physical dependence, which is the appearance of withdrawal symptoms when the drug is stopped suddenly. Pseudo addiction is a term that is used to describe behavior that appears "drug seeking" that is actually an effort to obtain relief. Tolerance is a state of adaptation in which exposure to a drug induces changes that result in a reduction of the drug's effects over time.

adjuvant. Drugs are used to strengthen the pain-relieving effect of opioids or to manage their side effects. This term is derived mainly from the cancer pain literature and includes medications such as tricycles antidepressants and anticonvulsants (used for neuropathic pain), which are now known to be true analgesics for certain types of pain.

allodynia. The presence of pain from a stimulus that is not normally painful. For example, pain from a sheet rubbing over the skin would be considered allodynia.

anergia. Lack of energy.

anhedonia. Psychological condition in which you stop enjoying things you previously enjoyed.

anticonvulsants. Medications used to treat seizures. Due to presumed common mechanisms underlying epilepsy and neuropathic pain, many anticonvulsants are effective in treating neuropathic pain.

antiemetic. Medication used for nausea and vomiting. Antiemetics improve a patient's ability to take medication for migraines by blocking the side effects.

biofeedback. Feedback from a device or computer to give information about physiological processes about which patients are not normally aware (e.g., muscle tension, skin temperature). Biofeedback may help relieve muscle tension caused by bracing muscles due to chronic pain.

breakthrough pain. An increase of pain beyond constant, background pain. Short-acting opioids are often prescribed for this purpose. One subcategory of breakthrough pain is "incident pain," which is pain that is provoked by certain "incidents," e.g. walking.

cancer pain. Pain associated with cancer, which can be the result of cancer itself or treatments for cancer (surgery, radiation, chemotherapy). It can be visceral, somatic, or neuropathic in nature.

central sensitization. Process by which pain is increased and maintained in the spinal cord or brain instead of being confined to other parts of the body. Central sensitization is thought to underlie some types of allodynia or hyperalgesia. It may also explain why surgically removing the "cause of the pain" may not eliminate the pain.

centralization. Loosely defined term that refers to the process by which a pain process that begins in the periphery, maintained by peripheral mechanisms, may over time become sustained partially or completely by central mechanisms. This concept overlaps with that of central sensitization. Centralization or central sensitization may also underlie evolution of the phenomenology of a chronic pain syndrome, such as the "spread" of reflex sympathetic dystrophy to other limbs.

chronic pain. Pain that persists over time beyond the expected healing period. Chronic pain can happen with many diseases, conditions, or injuries. Some sources define chronic pain as that persisting beyond three or six months after an injury.

cluster headaches. A strictly unilateral headache, usually occurring once or a few times a day at an uncharacteristic time (e.g. 1 AM), lasting for 15–180 minutes, occurring in a series which lasts for weeks to months, separated by remissions lasting from months to years. Cluster headaches are either episodic (described above) or chronic (without remission of at least 14 days). Cluster headaches usually occur on the same side of the head during a cluster period, but can shift from side to side in some patients.

cognitions. Thoughts. Cognitions can exert powerful effects on emotional reactions, responses and interpretations of pain on the patient.

cognitive-behavioral therapy. A form of psychological treatment that helps patients change their thoughts and behaviors to increase coping with pain, decrease negative affect, and increase functioning.

constipation. A condition in which bowel movements are infrequent or incomplete. This may be a complication of opiate pain medications.

de-education. See muscle de-education.

delirium. A syndrome characterized by combinations of cognitive deficits, fluctuating levels of consciousness, changes in sleep patterns, psychomotor agitation, hallucinations, delusions and/or perceptual abnormalities. Causes are multifactorial and can include psychotropic medications, opioids, metabolic changes, cancer treatment, sepsis, or brain tumor or metastases.

dependence. The symptoms of opiate withdrawal appear when the opiate is stopped suddenly. This happens to anyone taking daily opiates over several days. This is not a sign of addiction.

distraction. A pain coping technique that involves turning attention away from painful sensations.

dyspareunia. Pain during sex.

full or pure agonists. Opioids that block pain at nerve endings. There is no set maximum dose at which these medications will stop working. Examples include morphine, fentanyl, meperidine, codeine, and methadone.

heat. Refers to the application of heat via hot packs, hot water bottles, moist compresses, heating pads, chemical and gel packs, and immersion in water for the purpose of relief of pain.

hyperalgesia. The phenomenon whereby stimuli that are normally painful produce exaggerated pain. It can be ascertained by the response to single and multiple pinpricks on neurologic examination.

hyperpathia. A painful syndrome characterized by increased reaction to a stimulus, especially a repetitive stimulus, as well as increased threshold.

hypopathia. Refers to decreased responses to stimulation.

incident pain. Refers to the subset of breakthrough pain that is provoked by specific types of activity (e.g., walking, moving the arms).

long-acting opioids. An opioid with a relatively long duration of action. By tradition, opioids that last longer than about six to eight hours are referred to as long acting, but the border between short- and long-acting is not precise. Long-acting opioids may have a long duration by virtue of their intrinsic pharmacokinetics (e.g. methadone), by having been formulating in a tablet that delivers the medication over a long period of time (e.g. Kadian, Oxycontin), or by having been formulated in another type of delivery system (e.g. Duragesic patch). Several opioids are available in both short- and long-acting forms (e.g. morphine, oxycodone, fentanyl).

malingering. Involves the intentional production of false or grossly exaggerated physical or psychological symptoms for the purpose of tangible external incentives, such as obtaining financial compensation, evading criminal prosecution, avoiding work or military duty and obtaining drugs.

metabolite accumulation syndrome. Several opioids are metabolized to compounds that can accumulate and produce a characteristic syndrome. The features of this syndrome include anxiety, jitteriness, tremor, multifocal myoclonus, encephalopathy, convulsions, and death. This syndrome classically occurs with normeperidine, a metabolite of meperidine (Demerol), but has also been reported with morphine and hydromorphone. Other opioids have been reported to cause delirium and similar symptoms, but not due to metabolite accumulation, and without the other characteristic features noted above.

mixed agonists/antagonists. Opioids that block the pain-fighting ability of the pure agonist medications while providing pain relief at a different area on the nerve ending. These include nalbuphine (Nubain), pentazocine (Talwin), and butorphanol (Stadol).

modulation. The process of modification of nociceptive signals that takes place in the dorsal horn of the spinal cord and elsewhere with input from ascending and descending pathways.

multi-modal treatment. Treatment by more than one modality (i.e., physical therapy, medical, psychological).

muscle de-education. Occurs when pain or avoiding pain leads to the failure to activate muscles or the abnormal activation of muscles in movement.

neuropathic pain. Pain that is caused by a lesion in or dysfunction of the nervous system.

nociceptive pain. Pain that results from injury to or inflammation of somatic tissues.

nonpharmacologic treatment. Treatment that does not involve drugs (e.g, physical therapy, biofeedback, psychological treatment).

NSAIDS. A non-steroidal, anti-inflammatory drug. An aspirin-like drug used to reduce inflammation caused from injured tissue and pain. This includes aspirin and ibuprofen, but not acetaminophen.

Numerical Rating Scale (NRS). A method of rating pain intensity that involves written or verbal notation of pain on an 11–point scale by choosing a number from 0 (no pain) to 10 (pain as bad as it could be).

pain. An unpleasant sensory and emotional experience associated with actual or potential tissue damage or described in terms of such damage.

pain assessment. Evaluation of a variety of aspects of pain, including intensity, duration, frequency, description, location, and emotional responses, among others.

pain behaviors. Verbal or nonverbal expressions of pain including behavioral reactions, such as grimacing, rubbing the affected part, guarding or restriction of movement and sighing.

partial agonists. Opioid analgesics that produce analgesia by binding to the mu opioid receptor, but with less intrinsic efficacy at that receptor than "full agonists." These agents have a ceiling effect for analgesia and may precipitate withdrawal if administered to a physically dependent patient.

pathophysiology. The physiology of abnormal states.

peripheral sensitization. Process by which neurons in peripheral nerves become abnormally responsive to noxious or non-noxious stimuli, thereby facilitating exaggerated pain perception.

pharmacological treatment of chronic pain. Treatment of pain with medicine.

physical dependence. Is a state of adaptation that is manifested by a drug class specific withdrawal syndrome that can be produced by abrupt cessation, rapid, dose reduction, decreasing blood level of the drug, or administration of an antagonist.

physical therapy. Physical interventions, including passive modalities (i.e., application f heat and cold) and active modalities (e.g., range of motion, exercise) used to strengthen muscles, increase cardiovascular activity and restore normal functioning.

placebo. A harmless substance that has no active ingredient and no medication, like sterile water injection. Placebos are used in clinical trials to help show the effect of a medication.

primary afferent nociceptors. Pain receptors (A-delta or C fibers) that respond to noxious mechanical, thermal, and chemical stimuli.

primary headaches. Headaches that are autonomous without a specific lesion, whereas secondary headaches are connected to a specific lesion.

pseudo addiction. A term that is used to describe behavior that appears like addictive, "drug seeking" behavior but is actually an effort to obtain pain relief. Addictive behaviors are said to be distinguished from pseudo addiction when the behaviors resolve after treatment of pain.

referred pain. The perception of pain in parts of the body distant from the pathology from which the pain originates. Examples include arm pain during an acute myocardial infarction, or eye pain during vertebral artery dissection.

rest pain. Pain experienced while in an inactive or resting state.

secondary headaches. Headache associated with primary disease processes, such as brain tumors, head trauma, vascular disorders, and substance use and withdrawal.

somatoform disorder. An example of pain that is produced or amplified by psychological processes. Criteria are less restrictive than summarization disorder and require one or more physical complaints that cannot be explained by a general medical condition and cause significant social or occupational distress.

somatic pain. Refers to pain arising from somatic structures (e.g., skin, bones, muscle, joint). It is typically well-localized ("my left finger"), and worsened by pressure on, or movement of, the affected part.

somatization disorder. Psychological disorder characterized by a pattern of multiple physical complaints (e.g., pain symptoms, gastrointestinal symptoms, sexual problems) present before the age of 30 that causes significant social and occupational impairment.

stress management. Techniques designed to aid in the reduction of physiologic hyperarousal due to stress.

TENS. Transcutaneous Electrical Nerve Stimulation is a pain reduction technique that involves applying low-voltage electrical stimulation to the skin, stimulating large nerve fibers, and blocking other pain transmission.

tolerance. The need for an increased dose of opioid pain medication to get pain control. This can happen to anyone taking opioid medications and is not a sign of addiction.

transmission. The process by which nerve signals from the peripheral tissues are sent to the spinal cord.

tricyclic antidepressants. A class of antidepressants also used to assist the treatment of pain, sleep disturbance, and/or associated depressive symptoms.

visceral pain. Refers to pain arising from pathology of the visceral organs, such as bowel obstruction or pancreatitis. Such pain is typically poorly localized (e.g., my whole belly hurts) and is associated with visceral symptoms (e.g., nausea, vomiting).

Visual Analogue Scale (VAS). A method of measuring pain intensity that consists of a 10-centimeter line with anchors at the ends. Common anchors are "no pain" and "pain as bad as it could be." Patients draw a vertical line through the horizontal line and the result in centimeters is multiplied by 10, yielding a number between 0 and 100.

World Health Organization (WHO) ladder. Recommendations from the WHO for titration of therapy for cancer pain known as the "analgesic ladder." The ladder presents a three-step algorithm for using medications in the treatment of cancer pain, and includes five major treatment concepts: (1) by the mouth, (2) by the clock, (3) by the ladder, (4) for the individual, and (5) with attention to detail.

INDEX

non-medication treatments for, 149–150

Feverfew (herbal medicine), 126

Fentanyl (Duragesic, Sublimaze), 95

fibromyalgia, 34
  symptoms of, 34
  treatment for, 34

fun, therapeutic benefits of, 139–140

gabapentin (Neurontin), 82

gallbladder pain, 32

gallstones, 36, 58
  how formed, 36
  treatment for, 58

glucosamine (supplement), 128

gout, 24–25, 61
  treatment for, 25

head pain, 55–56

headaches, 29–31, 192
  causes of, 29–30
  migraines, 30–31, 55
  rebound headaches, 31
  tension or stress, 55–56

health care providers, 39–50
  doctor, 39–40
  finding the right, 44
  specialists, 40–44, 46

health care services
  cost of care, 46–47
  emergency rooms, 45–46
  insurance plans, 47–50
  pain clinics, 45

Healthy Diet Pyramid, 131–133, 137

heating pad, using for pain management, 97–98

hematologists, 40

hemophilia, 28–29, 98, 192

herbal medicines and supplements, 125–129
  capsaicin, 126–127
  chondrotin, 129
  Feverfew, 126
  glucosamine, 128
  magnetic therapy, 129
  St. John's Wort, 128
  willow bark, 127

herpes, 36

HIV and pain, 29

hospice care, 154–155
  and minorities, 7

hydrocodone, 88

hydromorphone (Dilaudid, Palladone), 88–89

hypnosis, for pain management, 112–113

ibuprofen, 78

imagery, using for pain management, 105–106

infections, 35, 60
  herpes, 36
  shingles, 35

inflammation and pain, 18–19
  NSAIDS and, 74–75
  steroids and, 74

inflammatory bowel disease, 32

injections (pain procedure), 118

injury and pain, 18
  treatment for, 24

insurance plans, 47–50

HMOs, 47–48
Medicare and Medicaid, 49–50
PPOs, 48–49
irritable bowel syndrome, 32

joint pain, 60–61. *See also* arthritis

Ketoprofen, 78
ketoralac (Toradol), 79–80
kidney stones, 33, 37, 59
    causes of, 59–60
    treatment for, 37, 59–60

levorphanol, 93–94
lidocaine (topical medication),
    72–73
LOCATES (medical history
    memory aid), 52–53, 67

magnetic therapy, 129
massage, using for pain management, 100
    therapeutic massage, 124–125
medical history, 51–53
    CT, MRI, thermography, 54–55
    lab work, 54
    LOCATES, 52–53
    physical examination, 53–54
    writing down your, 184–186
medical schools, teaching pain
    therapy, 150
medical services. *See* health care
    services
medical tests, 54–55
    blood tests, 61
    CAT Scan, 54, 56

MRI, 54, 56
    thermography, 54–55
Medicare and Medicaid, 49–50
    social security disability, 50,
        152–153
    web sites, 189–190
medications. *See* pain medications
meditation, for pain management, 107–108
meningitis, 55
Meperidine (Demerol), 90–91
    side effects, 91
methadone, 93–95
migraine headaches, 30. *See also*
    headaches
    causes of, 30–31, 55
    infections associated with,
        30–31
    medications for, 30
    symptoms of, 21
    triggers for, 55
mind/body therapies, 105–116
    distraction, 114–116, 139
    hypnosis, 111–113
    imagery, 105–106
    meditation, 107–108
    prayer, 108–111
    relaxation therapy, 106–107
    spiritual life, 140–141
    yoga, 113–114
minorities, and pain, 145, 150
    hospice care, 7
mood changes, keeping track of,
    64
morphine, 91–93
    capsules, 92

massage, 100
therapeutic ultrasound, 98–99
transcutaneous electrical nerve
stimulation, 101–102
physician assistants (PAs), 42
podiatrists, 40
prayer, using for pain management, 108–111
Bible scriptures, 108–111
primary-care doctor, 186
propoxyphene (Darvon), 96
psychiatrists and psychologists,
42

radiologists, 40
relaxation therapy, for pain management, 106–107
techniques, 106, 107
resources
books, 206–207
glossary, 209–219
pain assessment tools, 180–186
web sites, 187–206
rheumatologists, 40, 46

salicylate salts, 73
shingles (Herpes Zoster), 35, 58
treatment for, 35, 72
sickle cell disease, 28, 192, 197
treatment for, 28
sinus infections, 56
sleep, 138–139
rest breaks, 139
social security disability benefits,
50, 152–153
social workers, 42–43
spinal stenosis, 60

spiritual life, 140–141
prayer, 108–111
St. John's Wort (herbal medicine), 128
statistics on pain, 4–6
steroids, 74
stress, and back pain, 56
stretching of organs, 20
sub-acute pain, 16
support groups, 141, 197
surgeons, 40
surgery, for pain relief, 119

TMJ (temporomandibular joint)
pain, 27
topical pain medications, 72–73
Tramadol (Ultram), 83
transcutaneous electrical nerve
stimulation (TENS), 101–102
tumors and infections, 60

ulcers, 58
ultrasound, therapeutic, 98–99
benefits of, 98–99
how it works, 99
urologists, 41

visceral pain, 20
vitamins, daily, 136
vocational rehabilitation, 43–44

web sites, 194–206
clinical trials, 187–189
clinics, 197
disease specific, 191–192
drugs, 190–191
end of life pain, 194